THE
DISTANT HEALING
HANDBOOK

Also by Jack Angelo

Your Healing Power: A comprehensive guide to channelling your healing energies

The Spiritual Healing Handbook: How to develop your healing powers and increase your spiritual awareness

(with Jan Angelo)

About the Author

Jack Angelo has been a teacher and writer in the fields of energy medicine and natural spirituality since the mid 1980s. His work as a healer began when he intuitively sent healing to others. Since then he has developed Distant Healing – a comprehensive healing method based on his research and work with individuals and groups in the UK and abroad. For 10 years Jack was a tutor with the NFSH. Having worked with American Indian medicine teachers, Jack sees indigenous and shamanic wisdom as the origin of all spiritual traditions and a gateway through which we can access healing and spirituality. His books have been translated into 16 languages.

THE DISTANT HEALING HANDBOOK

How to send healing to people, animals, the environment and global trouble spots

JACK ANGELO

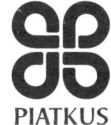
PIATKUS

Visit the Piatkus website!

Piatkus publishes a wide range of bestselling fiction and non-fiction, including books on health, mind, body & spirit, sex, self-help, cookery, biography and the paranormal.

If you want to:
- read descriptions of our popular titles
- buy our books over the internet
- take advantage of our special offers
- enter our monthly competition
- learn more about your favourite Piatkus authors

VISIT OUR WEBSITE AT: www.piatkus.co.uk

Copyright © 2007 by Jack Angelo

First published in Great Britain in 2007 by
Piatkus Books Ltd
5 Windmill Street, London W1T 2JA
email: info@piatkus.co.uk

The moral right of the author has been asserted

A catalogue record for this book is available from the British Library

ISBN 9 780 7499 2815 5

Text design by Paul Saunders
Edited by Anthea Matthison

This book has been printed on paper manufactured
with respect for the environment using wood from
managed sustainable resources

Typeset by Phoenix Photosetting, Chatham, Kent
www.phoenixphotosetting.co.uk

Printed and bound in Great Britain by
Mackays of Chatham, Chatham, Kent

Acknowledgements

My thanks to: all the workshop participants and all those I have sent out to over the years – you are a vital part of this book; Jan Angelo, for her support and inspiration; Elspeth Samuel who rescued me from computer failure; Judy Piatkus, Gill Bailey and the team at Piatkus Books for their great help in making it possible to give this book to the world; and Rob Hume, editor of *Birds,* for permission to quote from the article mentioned in Chapter 11.

Contents

Acknowledgements — v
The exercises — ix
Illustrations — xiii
Introduction — 1

Part One

1 Widening our circle of compassion — 11
2 Your healing hands — 20
3 Your light body — 27
4 Preparations for getting started — 35
5 Baseline practice — 51
6 Baseline practice – the healing circle — 61

Part Two

7 The energy circuits of the body — 71
8 Etheric gateways – the subtle energy centres — 81
9 Addressing the effects of personal feelings and negative energies — 99
10 Advanced Distant Healing — 113

Part Three

11 Working with the environment — 133

12 Working with plants and animals — 149

13 Taking action to heal local and global issues — 165

Part Four

14 A way of being — 179

Glossary — 193

Further reading — 196

Web resources — 198

Index — 201

The exercises

Part One

1 Widening our circle of compassion — 11
   1 Attunement — 17

2 Your healing hands — 20
   2 Activating the palm centres — 21
   3 Sensing the quality of your hands' energies — 21
   4 Sensing the energies of a partner's hands — 22
   5 Breathing energy into the hands — 23
   6 Sending out energy from your hands — 24
   7 Sending energy to a partner — 25

3 Your light body — 27
   8 Sensing the energy field — 30
   9 Sensing information in the energy field — 32

4 Preparations for getting started — 35
   10 Clearing the energy field — 37
   11 The Rainbow Breath — 39
   12 Full-breath breathing — 43
   13 Full-body relaxation — 45
   14 Preparing and dedicating the work space — 48

5 Baseline practice — 51
- 15 Sending out the healing Light — 54
- 16 Creating the Light pool — 55
- 17 Regulating the energy centres — 58
- 18 The Sphere of Protection — 59

6 Baseline practice – the healing circle — 61
- 19 The Distant Healing Circle – sending out the healing Light — 62
- 20 The Distant Healing Circle – creating the Light column — 64

Part Two

7 The energy circuits of the body — 71
- 21 Sensing the skeletal energy circuits — 75
- 22 Sensing the skeletal energy circuits – partner on a chair — 77
- 23 Checking polarity balance — 78
- 24 Checking polarity balance – partner on a chair — 79

8 Etheric gateways – the subtle energy centres — 81
- 25 Sensing the location of the centres — 83
- 26 Sensing Earth energies with the Sole-of-the-Foot Centres — 96
- 27 Sensing the hand-heart energy circuit — 97

9 Addressing the effects of personal feelings and negative energies — 99
- 28 Body awareness — 108
- 29 Accessing body secrets — 109
- 30 Working with your feelings — 110

10 Advanced distant healing — 113
- 31 Astral level healing — 117
- 32 The astral level Healing Circle – with one joint list — 122
- 33 The astral level Healing Circle – with individual lists — 125

Part Three

11 Working with the environment — 133
   34 Communing with the Earth — 138
   35 Communing with Water — 140
   36 Communing with Fire — 140
   37 Communing with Air — 141
   38 Engaging with your landscape — 143
   39 Responding to an environmental issue – sending out healing Light — 145
   40 Responding to an environmental issue – creating the Light pool — 146

12 Working with plants and animals — 149
   41 Engaging with the plant world — 151
   42 Listening to a tree — 152
   43 Sending Distant Healing to the plant world — 152
   44 Communing with the animal realm — 156
   45 Working with a sick animal – astral level healing — 158
   46 Sending healing to a dying animal — 161
   47 Creating the Light pool for a dying animal — 162
   48 Telling your Earth story — 163

13 Taking action to heal local and global issues — 165
   49 Sending Light into a locality — 167
   50 Sending Light to a disaster situation – the Distant Healing Circle — 169
   51 Sending out to the injured and dying – astral level healing — 172

Part Four

14 A way of being — 179
   52 Assessing the state of the heart centre — 180
   53 Heart centre breathing — 182

54 Balancing body energies	183
55 The Seven Breaths of Greeting	185
56 Blessing and thanking food	186
57 Sending out to a project	188
58 Honouring beauty and the natural world	190

Illustrations

1	The Healing Triangle	12
2	Sensing your hands' energies	22
3	Breathing energy into the hands	24
4	Sending out energy from the hands	25
5	The human energy field	29
6	Sensing the energy field	31
7	The etheric body and the seven main energy centres	33
8	Clearing the energy field	38
9	The Rainbow Breath	40
10	How breathing works	42
11	The Sphere of Protection	59
12	The Distant Healing Circle – creating the Light column	66
13	The polarity channels of the etheric body	72
14	The skeletal energy circuits	74
15	The seven main energy centres and the centres of the hands and feet	82
16	Sensing the crown centre	84
17	Sensing the brow centre	85
18	Sensing the base centre	86
19	The energy field of the astral body	116
20	Astral level healing	119
21	Astral level healing – the Sphere of Protection	120
22	The astral level Healing Circle	123
23	A disrupted landscape	144
24	A disaster situation	169

THE
DISTANT HEALING
HANDBOOK

Introduction

LOVE IS AN ENERGY with the power to unite, harmonise and heal, and it is unconditional in its action. Distant Healing is the transmission of this energy, through a person's desire and intention to help, to where it is needed. Instead of being present, as in hands-on healing or other forms of energy therapy, the subject is at some distance from us – hence 'distant healing'. (When Distant Healing appears with capitals it refers to the special method and techniques described in this book.)

The great advantage of this form of healing is that the 'subject' can be a person, an animal, a plant, an environment and even a situation. This book explains how this works, how to do it, what happens during the process, and the different ways in which it can used. These range from working with friends and family, pets and the home, to the environment, societal and global problems. The book is accessible, at a number of levels, to anyone interested in healing energies and to all those who want to work with them. This includes beginners, as well as practising energy workers, therapists and health-care professionals.

The Distant Healing perspective

From the Distant Healing perspective, healing energies come from the Source of all energy – a Oneness which religious people call God. The energies thus originate *outside* the space-time frame of the physical level and so they are not governed by its laws until they enter this level. This means that they can travel to another person, another being, landscape, or situation, at any distance from us, in an instant.

Why Distant Healing?

There are factors and situations where hands-on help is just not possible. For example, distance prevents certain people from travelling. This is the case with the disabled, those in some kind of confinement, those with a mental or behavioural condition, the sick, and of course those who live just too far away. As a Distant Healer, none of these factors presents a barrier to your being able to offer help.

Similarly, because it is able to work at an energetic level with the energies involved, Distant Healing is an ideal way to address the two urgent issues of our time – environmental and societal problems, whether local or global.

The feeling that you want to help another, or do something about a situation, is the instinct to heal. When people ask me if they need special qualifications to work as a Distant Healer, I assure them that the most important qualification is this instinct – which comes from the heart.

The instinct to heal

I have always been fascinated by the fact that people in all cultures throughout recorded time have been laying hands on others to ease pain, relieve symptoms, and often to completely heal a condition. This is not surprising when you consider that when we hurt ourselves our first instinct is to immediately send unconscious thoughts of healing to the place that hurts by putting our hands on it. When this happens to us as children our mother opens her arms to cuddle us and 'kiss it better'. This instinct is a loving gesture which comes before any rational thought of what to do about it. You don't need to think about how to be loving or supportive, you just do it.

In the mid 1980s, I was 'encouraged' to discover what this meant in practice. Months of chronic back trouble and sciatica had baffled my doctor and he suggested that I visit a healer. 'After all,' he said, 'what have you got to lose?' The upshot was that my back trouble was considerably improved and I pondered on how it was done. But my visits had convinced me that I already knew how it was done. I had been 'doing it' for others since I was a child.

Discovering subtle energies

My encounter with this healer proved to be life changing. I was a curious patient and Dennis, my healer, did his best to answer my questions but assured me that I would make my own discoveries. This launched me into the world of healing and subtle energy medicine – the therapies that work with 'subtle' energies. Subtle energies travel at speeds beyond the speed of light and so are not visible to normal sight and everyday sensing. Because of this, some people have found this fact of life difficult to understand or accept.

But I had been aware of these energies ever since I could remember – sometimes I 'saw' them and, more often than not, I sensed them in some other way. For example, I saw light round people. When they were angry or unhappy this light became frighteningly dark. When I sat with old people my hands would sometimes tingle or get warm. To me, this type of awareness was quite normal and I assumed that everyone was like me. As I grew up, I discovered that we all have the natural ability to sense subtle energies, even if we don't exercise it. It is exciting to realise that healing energies fall into this category. They are subtle, but they can certainly be sensed or felt by most of us.

The healer described his work as the action of love. This was an energy that came from the Source, 'through' him and into the patient. It was love that did the healing. But he saw this as complementary to everyday medicine not as an alternative or last resort for the desperate. Dennis's assertion that love could heal did not sound corny to me – it sounded obvious. But I had never heard any sort of therapy described in this way before.

Healing at a distance

Quite soon after my time with Dennis, I had the chance to consider his point of view, and to put it into practice, on a trip to Italy. Readers of *Your Healing Power* may recall this story. I repeat it here because it tells how I started distant healing and how, in this field of therapy, you can expect the unexpected. I spent my first night in the beautiful Tuscan town of San Gimignano in a family home. As I lay awake planning the research I was to do in the coming month, little did I know that I was beginning a life in healing. The house had been quiet for some time when suddenly a rasping sound broke the silence. Grandfather Fanciulli was coughing. On and on he coughed until the coughs changed to groans and cries of desperation. But the rest of the house remained still. No one went to his aid. Perhaps the family slept through it because they were already used to these harrowing sounds and felt powerless to bring him any form of relief.

I wanted to help him. I was lying on my back and something made me put my hands outside the bedclothes as if I could send some 'healing' towards the grandfather. To my surprise, my palms and fingertips began tingling – a feeling at once strange yet oddly familiar. I mentally asked for help to be sent to the old man. The next moment his coughing stopped abruptly. The house returned to silence and I dropped off to sleep.

In the small hours of the next night the old man began to cough again, hardly able to pause for breath, until it sounded as if he would cough up his whole body. There was no space for a groan or a cry. Again I stretched out my hands and asked for help for him, and again his coughing stopped immediately.

The same thing happened every night until I left San Gimignano. As I said goodbye to the Fanciullis, old Nonno gave me a smile which seemed to say that he knew what had been happening. Perhaps on some level he did know, but this first attempt at distant healing taught me that whatever was making my hands tingle could be sent somewhere to help. I did not need to analyse how this could happen. During the rest of my time in Italy I frequently felt the need to send healing thoughts out to people I passed in the street. I guessed that this was healing at a distance, distant healing, and it seemed such an easy way to help out.

Working as a Distant Healer

On my return to my home in Wales, the locality of a small mining village seemed a daunting place when faced with what needed to be done. The land and the people were trying to recover from centuries of mining and now from the trauma of closure and unemployment. A clever, mocking voice in my head seemed to be saying, 'Come on, Jack. What can you do here with distant healing?' Something needed to happen to balance my innate scepticism. I joined a local meditation group. The leader said she sensed that I had the gift of healing and suggested I send distant healing to a list of people she had drawn up. She did not tell me how to do this, saying that I would be 'inspired from within' to find my own way intuitively.

One evening after a meeting of the group a young woman came up to me. She was obviously pregnant. She had heard I was a healer and wondered if I could help her. Her boyfriend had left her, her parents had thrown her out of their home, and the foetus kept returning to the breech position, no matter how many times it was turned by the midwife. Without wondering how, I said I would do my best. I would work out what that would be later. That night I sat quietly in a chair. Using my breathing to help me relax, I attuned to the Source. When I felt centred, I asked if I could help the young woman.

With closed eyes, I soon sensed the body of a woman as if it was laid out in front of me, hovering in mid-air. Instead of being surprised, I assumed this was part of the process and relied on my instinct to heal. My palms were already tingling. As I reached out, I could 'feel' her baby in the womb, and other unknown hands gently turned it so that the head faced downwards again. This was accompanied by an overwhelming sense that everything would be all right for mother and baby. I sat for a while, just absorbing the experience. Suddenly the feeling came to 'hand over' their fate to the higher power that seemed to be looking after them. I got up and thought no more about it.

I didn't see the young woman for a while. Then a few months later she turned up at the group meeting again. She had a few things to report. Her baby boy did not return to the breech position and was born naturally. Her boyfriend came to her hospital bedside and asked her to marry him. 'What wonderful news!' I said. But that wasn't all. Her parents seemed to have had a change of heart too because they also visited her and welcomed her back to their home. I heard the list in amazement. So this was the world of distant healing!

Sometimes I sent help and nothing seemed to happen. I had to learn not to take it personally when people didn't bother to report back one way or the other. But during the ensuing weeks positive feedback from many of those who had requested my help gave me proof that distant healing was effective for all kinds of conditions.

Becoming aware of the energies

When I sat to do distant healing, I was aware of an energetic change in my hands which would be the signal that I was working. But this was not always accompanied by a sense of the presence of the person who needed the help. When this did happen, I was able to sense the body from whatever angle seemed necessary. I knew where on the body I needed to place my hands and the organs concerned gave off information about what was wrong. I often 'saw' or 'felt' what was taking place as the healing progressed. In this way I was able to work with people as if they were physically present. I also picked up a range of messages coming from different parts of a person's body. These told not only of the physical conditions, but of worries, sadness, stress, past traumas, life incidents, unfulfilled needs, as if everything that had happened to that person was recorded somewhere in the body or in the energy field of that body.

Part One of this book will prepare you for experiences like these and in Part Two we will look at them in detail to see how they can contribute to more advanced work.

My healing journey

My journey into healing began with distant healing. I kept a working journal and built up a very useful database of experience which gave me an excellent grounding and understanding when I came to work 'hands on'. My interest in the natural world led me to work with the healing ways of many indigenous peoples, especially the Native Americans. Even though I was only able to work with these 'medicine' people for a few days at a time, I found that they were able to transmit further teachings at a distance. Sometimes I would wake up and grab paper and pencil, realising I had just been instructed during my sleep. As well as years of workshop experience, this book also includes the knowledge gained from my indigenous, or 'shamanic' encounters.

During 25 years of 'hands-on' subtle energy work I have written a number of books on the subject, including *Your Healing Power*, which has become an international healing classic. Its sequel, *The Spiritual Healing Handbook*, will appeal to those who want to take the work even further.

Things have come full circle and distant healing is again my main therapeutic focus.

The next step for healers – Distant Healing

The dozen or so years since *Your Healing Power* was published, in 1994, have prepared those who have used my books for the next important step in healing. This is to work with those situations where hands-on healing is difficult or impossible. This field of work has been considerably expanded now that two further, but crucial, issues present themselves. Their call to us is urgent and, like the child who has fallen over and lies crying, there is little time for us to stop and think about what to do. These issues concern our global environment, the Earth, and the fear which fuels chaos and violence everywhere on this beautiful planet. This is why this book is needed now.

How to use the book

Start your practice, like I did, by learning how to send out to another person, or a favourite pet. With exercises at each stage, the book will guide you carefully, giving you a firm foundation from which you can move on to the more advanced work in Part Two. Stay with each section until you feel confident with the practice.

You will have many experiences once you start work and Chapters 7, 8 and 9 are designed to prepare you for them. You can start your Distant Healing work straight away and dip into these when you feel the need. Keep a journal of your progress. This will help you to build your own database of experience.

About the exercises

The exercises are designed to lead you to the point where you will feel confident to begin making Distant Healing a life skill. The exercises with a partner are essential for developing your knowledge base, but not essential to your work as a caring individual. Your knowledge base can be acquired over time by practice when the opportunity arises.

You may find it helpful to record some of the exercises so that you can be free to carry them out without referring back to the book. Or your working partner could read them out for you.

Interaction with a partner or a group brings the extra dimension of being with others which is so helpful in developing an open and compassionate heart. But there may be reasons why you have to work on your own. When this is the case, it is worth recalling that you care about others because you are aware of them and their needs, and you are aware of being part of a diverse global family. Through Distant Healing, you essentially interact with others so that you are an effective and vital contributor to individual and world healing.

Meanwhile, it is important not to let your lack of a working partner stop you from making a start with Distant Healing. You will soon see that the exercises for individual practice will prepare you to work quite adequately.

Practise the exercises and experiment with the techniques in the book to find out how Distant Healing works. Keeping a journal will allow you to maintain your own record of what you do and the results that you observe. Sooner or later a pattern will emerge that will indicate that you are creating your own individual practice.

Please note that none of the exercises should be used for purposes other than those specified.

Part One

Chapter 1

Widening our circle of compassion

What is Distant Healing?

For millennia, healing at a distance has been a time-honoured way of ministering to the sick and needy. Evidence from around the world shows that this form of healing has always been just as common as hands-on healing. Among the Middle Eastern peoples of the first century CE, for example, two famous healers from Galilee are recorded as working this way: in the healing of the great Gamli'el's son by Hanina ben Dosa (in *Babylonian Talmud: Berakhot 34b*) and the healing of the royal official's son by Yeshua/Jesus (in *John 4: 46–53*).

People with different world views or religious beliefs have different ways of defining distant healing, explaining how it works and the energies that they are working with. Moreover, each world view has a different *language* to describe the process. At an individual level, people's life experience and their at-onement with their own life journey all influence these views and definitions. However, all world views understand the instinct to offer help to another. We can do this by thought, by what we say and what we do.

Your instinct to heal means that you may have often sent out a thought or prayer that healing will be directed to a person, animal, the environment or a situation. In Distant Healing, we further strengthen this simple, but loving, impulse with the power of spiritual intention. Here, the Distant Healer is able to both channel and transmit healing energies through conscious attunement to the Source of these energies.

How Distant Healing works – the Healing Triangle

In the first stage of Distant Healing, we attune to, or align ourselves with, the source of all energy – Oneness. This can happen in a variety of ways, from being in nature, to 'losing ourselves' in a creative task, to the simple method I outline in the first exercise, on page 17. You will know when this has happened. You will sense it as a feeling of being centred and serene, relaxed yet alert. Once you are attuned, you are in a state of readiness to create the links that allow healing energy to flow.

When you form your healing intention, to send out to a loved one say, you make an energetic link with that person. This, in turn, opens up the link between your loved one (the subject) and the Source. You have effectively set up what I call the Healing Triangle.

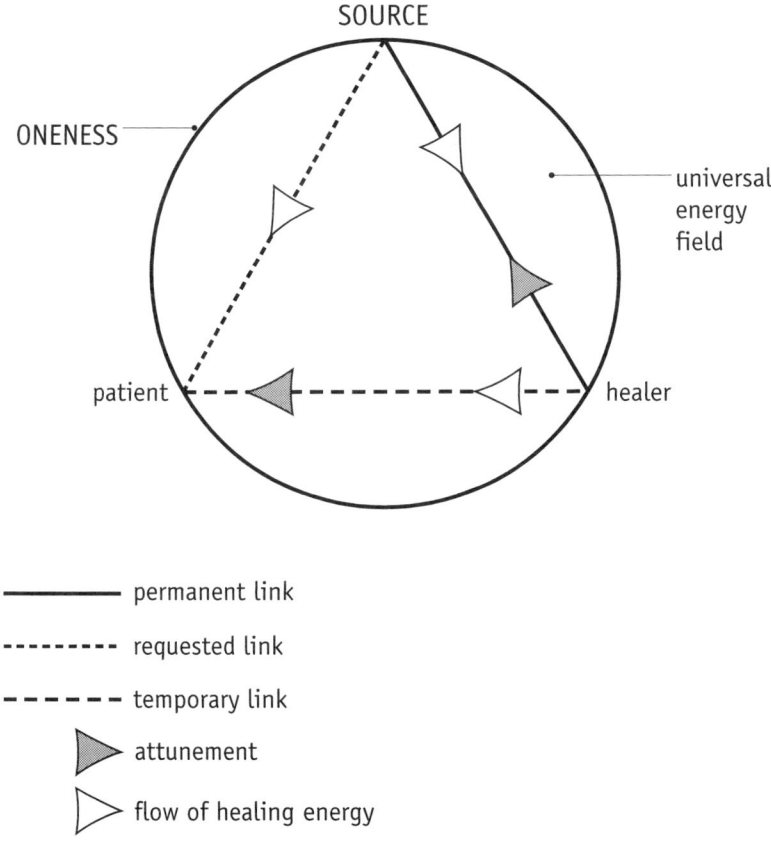

Figure 1. The Healing Triangle

This bridges the spiritual level, from where healing energies originate, and the physical level of the space-time frame, where they are needed. The 'subject' in the Healing Triangle is the person, animal, place or situation you wish to work with. When you link with the subject you activate the link between the subject and the Source. In the illustration, the Triangle is set within a circle to signify the oneness of all three points and the dedicated protective circle you will be working with. By creating the Healing Triangle, distance is overcome, for love energy has the power to travel both outside and inside the boundaries of space and time.

The healing process begins at the spiritual level. From here it travels 'downwards' to the other levels of being. This means that energy will sometimes reach the physical instantly and bring about change, but sometimes energy will be needed on a subtle level first (such as the mental, for example) and change will be seen more slowly on the physical. These things depend on the cause (or causes) of the condition, the soul's journey and the state of readiness of a person. This can involve the balancing factors of the law of cause and effect. When souls decide to address imbalances created in the present life, or in past lives, the factors of this law will influence the energetic situation.

The power of intention

It has been shown by many researchers, including Dr Larry Dossey, that intentionality has a bearing on the outcome of the energetic process (see Further Reading and Web Resources, pages 196 and 198). For this reason, the request is made unconditionally so that healing is directed to where it is needed and not necessarily how we, with our limited knowledge, think it should be applied. In other words we simply ask for healing to be sent, without limiting our request to a specific condition. For example, it is more appropriate to ask: 'May healing be sent to (name),' rather than 'Please cure her cancer'.

This acknowledges the fact that a person is a spiritual being and that it is the spirit that dictates the activities of the healing force. It also honours the soul's evolutionary journey and deeper reason for a condition about which we actually know nothing. This attitude does not see health as an isolated condition of the body. Instead, we co-operate with the body consciousness, rather than manipulate it.

Distant Healing, loss and illness

As well as those situations where hands-on healing is either not possible or inappropriate, Distant Healing always helps a person to pass over – to let go of the body. In responding to a request for help over a passing, or terminal illness, the Distant Healer is joining the person on this part of their journey. In the case of sudden death, through accident or injury, this help is invaluable. Healing can also be sent to the bereaved and anyone else affected by the death. There is always a team of people involved in a passing and the team will benefit from the healing you send to it.

People may also request help over an illness or operation. Here again, the Distant Healer is joining the person on this part of their journey. Those supporting ill or disabled people will also benefit from your healing help. And, just as in the bereavement situation, there is always a team involved in an illness or operation. Distant Healing will ensure that the team will receive the energetic boost it needs to do its best for the patient.

The challenge of the global community

We are part of a global community and our relationship with all life on planet Earth becomes evident when news of every distressing event around the world finds its way into our home. Many feel powerless in the face of this information onslaught. While enriching our lives with useful knowledge, the media at the same time have become a source of fear, telling us that life is not safe any more. We feel that we could do without their constant reminders about crime, societal breakdown and environmental disaster. As unknown others seem to take charge of our lives, our experience as separate from each other and from everything else is heightened.

We have to find ways to cope with these stresses and the most common response is to 'switch off', to become apathetic or even cynical. Switching off can be finding something to make us feel good for a while. There are plenty of those distractions, and it's easy to become addicted to some of them. On the other hand, if we are pessimistic we won't be constantly disappointed. Unfortunately, coping strategies like these only encourage us to live in fear.

In the last century, the celebrated physicist and Nobel Prize winner, Albert Einstein, forced by persecution to flee from Germany to Britain and then America, understood such feelings. A letter he wrote in 1950 shows that he recognised that most of us, though being part of a spiritual whole, nevertheless experience a deep sense of separation from everything and everyone else. But, Einstein insisted, we can break free from these feelings by widening 'our circle of compassion to embrace all living creatures and the whole of nature in its beauty'.

This phrase resonates with me as a description of Distant Healing for, as well as embracing the traditional role of reaching out to the sick and needy, the new agenda of Distant Healing widens 'our circle of compassion' to address the urgent problems of our time. This form of compassionate action is a spiritual activity that strengthens and maintains our spiritual core.

Distant Healing – an essential life skill

Our reconnection with the sacred gives progressively more meaning to life, and our part in it, and provides the foundations for a sustainable civilisation. As Distant Healing enlarges the traditional role of healing, it emerges as an essential life skill for all those who wish to bring harmony and well-being to the twenty-first century.

For practising healers and therapists already making a contribution, this book will provide a wider context and will enhance practice. However, you don't have to be a trained therapist to participate – you just have to want to.

A way into healing

Distant Healing could be your way back to empowerment and a way into helping or healing; it may become an important addition to your therapeutic repertoire; or it may become the healing practice that you prefer. It will always be a source of self-discovery as well as revealing how healing works. Distant Healing allows you to work quietly and anonymously or it can introduce you to a world, people and situations you would never have met otherwise – it's your choice.

You will find that you do not need to go looking for people or places to 'heal'. The law of attraction means that people will seek your help because the time is right for both of you to meet, as your individual paths cross. The meeting has a sacred dimension since it has been 'arranged' at a soul level with the agreement of all concerned. In this way, Distant Healing can help to heal the world as well as people, heal the landscape as well as animals and plants, heal situations as well as conditions. Your heart will direct you and show you how to heal the place that hurts, whatever form that 'place' may take.

Trusting your experience

My Distant Healing experiences are also part of my own spiritual journey. Your experiences will be unique to you and should be treated as such. There are few rules and norms in subtle energy work apart from attuning to the Source of healing, realising that all with whom you will work are a manifestation of that Oneness, and to work from the heart. In this way you will be guided by your inner self to the methods that are best for you. If you observe what happens and keep a careful record, it will become your own database. You will learn what you need to learn and do what you need to do. It is important to keep an open mind because your inner promptings may be to work with other beings and situations that you might not have otherwise considered.

Sooner or later you will be faced with the question: is it right to send help to those who have not requested it? You will have to make your own decision. I have found that a good strategy, whenever any decision has to be made, is to ask your heart: What would love do? My own answer is that love would want to help in some way. I also know that, because healing energies first engage with the *soul* concerned, that soul can decide whether or not to accept them. If they are rejected they simply pass on to where they can do some good. So nothing is lost.

In my own practice over the years, I have met very few of the people with whom I have worked. Many live on the other side of the world. Most often I receive a request for help from someone close to the person concerned. In those cases I always ask for feedback to be given on a regular basis so that I know how the person is progressing. Even so, you can be sure that people forget to do this and you can be left wondering how they are. This is why I find it most helpful to do my best and then leave it in the capable hands of the spiritual powers concerned, without giving the work any further thought.

Attunement

Since Distant Healing is about taking action, let's pause at this point to take stock and try the first exercise, which is about the experience of attunement, or alignment with the Source. This can be carried out indoors or outdoors.

EXERCISE 1

Attunement

Recall that attunement for Distant Healing is aligning your individual self with the Higher Self, or soul, and with the energies of healing. This consists of effective posture, effective breathing, relaxed awareness and focus. You will need to bring your focus to your *heart centre*. This is the subtle energy centre in the middle of your chest. We will study this energy centre in detail later. For now, think of it as the 'place' where your soul, or Higher Self, takes up residence.

First, notice how you are sitting and how you are breathing. Are you aware of anything going on around you? These awarenesses will soon become second nature once you begin practising the exercises.

The way we breathe and the way we use our breath is the key to how we energise ourselves. It even affects the way we think. Our breathing, in turn, is influenced by our posture. From here on we'll choose the best posture for relaxed, but effective, breathing. This will ensure effective energy circulation.

In all the exercises, 'relaxed' never means slumped or stooped. Relaxed means without tension, hanging loose, while remaining alert in your attention to the world.

- Sit well back in your chair, or cross-legged on the ground, so that the two girdles of the pelvis and shoulders are in line. Your

exercise continues ▶

spine should be straight, without pushing the chest forward. Hold your head up without straining. Rest your hands, palms up, on your thighs. Have your feet flat on the floor, feeling your connection with the ground. This is your connection with the Earth.

- Now close your eyes, while remaining totally alert. Using your breath, relax your body. With each out-breath relax your pelvis, feeling yourself sinking into the chair. Relax your shoulders and the back of your neck.

- Breathe naturally, through the nose. Your mouth is lightly closed with the jaws unclenched. Your tongue will settle into its own position, but you can begin by putting the front of your tongue against the hard palate, just behind your top front teeth.

- Breathe gently into your abdomen and enjoy the feeling of being relaxed and yet alert. Whenever you take up the sitting posture, this is the state you will need to achieve.

- Bring your focus to your heart centre. Now, relaxed, but fully aware, and breathing naturally, allow yourself to be at one with your Higher Self. Spend a few moments in union with Oneness, recalling that your Higher Self (or soul) is at one with the Source.

- Allow all thoughts to pass through your mind unobstructed. Any sounds around you are simply the accompaniment to your attunement. You are in the world. Nothing disturbs you. You are at one with the Source (or whatever is your concept of the Source).

- Give thanks to the Source for the opportunity to be used as a channel for healing. Ask to be as pure a channel as possible. Ask for protection for yourself and all the people, other beings, situations, you will be engaging with. Dedicate yourself and your work and ask for it to be blessed. Add any other prayers you wish, aware that you and the Source are one.

Aids to attunement

Your attunement, with your focus in the heart centre, will be the key element in all your Distant Healing work. Since attunement means aligning yourself with the sacred, use whatever helps you to arrive at that state. Dedicating and preparing your work space will begin the process, but you may find things like lighting incense, listening to music, sitting in front of your shrine, chanting, prayer, using musical instruments, or a short meditation, can all be means to achieve alignment. I find that, when I am outdoors, the mere presence of the natural world helps me to attune very quickly. Experiment to find out what works for you.

Through conscious attunement you make your link with your Higher Self and the source of healing energies. As I described earlier, this activates the first side of a very powerful energetic structure – the Healing Triangle. When you link with the subject to whom you are going to send Distant Healing, you activate the second side. This, in turn, opens up the subject's own link with the Source to activate the third side of the Healing Triangle.

When I began Distant Healing, I knew I was in an attuned state of readiness because of what my hands were telling me. We may be at a distance from our subject, but our hands still have an important role to play in the work. This is because they have a direct energetic link with our heart centre. In the next chapter we'll build on the experience of attunement to discover the role of the hands in Distant Healing.

Chapter 2

Your healing hands

IN THIS CHAPTER, you are going to become acquainted with your *healing* hands. This begins a new relationship with your hands which will continue to develop as you work your way through the book.

Our hands always let us know how we feel in our heart. If we love someone, the chances are that we will want to touch them. Pet owners reinforce the bond with their furry friends by stroking them. Yet the urge to use our hands to hurt is a sure indicator that we have lost contact with love and affection.

Healing teaches that there is an energetic link between the hands and the heart and, although Distant Healing begins with thought and intention, our hands become a useful guide when we are working this way. They lead us to the place where healing energy is needed because they have a subtle sensing apparatus which is sensitive to energy flow and imbalance. If we co-operate with it, this sensing mechanism is activated and guided by the power of intuition – a faculty of our Higher Self. If you practise allowing the sensitivity of your hands to work in tandem with your intuition, they will prove to be a guide and helper you can trust.

It is possible to activate the subtle sensing centres of your palms. They have a direct link with the heart energy centre and activation helps prepare the hands for any subtle or therapeutic work, including Distant Healing. So we begin our new relationship with the hands with a simple exercise.

EXERCISE 2
Activating the palm centres

- First, take a good look at your hands. Turn them over slowly so that you see both sides as well as the surfaces of the back of the hand and the palms. Try to look at them as if you are seeing them for the first time. These are your tools for reaching out and helping others.

- Now close both hands to make a loose fist, squeezing the tips of the fingers against the palms. Squeeze and let go. Do this a number of times in rapid succession until both hands feel energised.

- The same result may be achieved by gently rubbing the palms together in a circular motion. You may feel a tingling or warmth in your palms. Remember this sensation.

With this next simple activation exercise, you are ready to get to know how your hands react to subtle energies.

EXERCISE 3
Sensing the quality of your hands' energies

- Stand or sit comfortably. Take three full breaths into the abdomen to energise yourself.

- Hold your hands up to about waist height, with your palms facing inwards, and the width of your body between them. Let the hands relax so that the fingers separate naturally. Notice what you sense between your two palms.

- Bring your hands together slowly, again noticing what you sense as you do so.

exercise continues ▶

- Try again with the hands stretched a little wider apart, this time being aware of the energies like strands of elastic stretching from hand to hand.

- Vary the distance between your hands. Turn them over. Move your hands together in different ways. Note the various sensations.

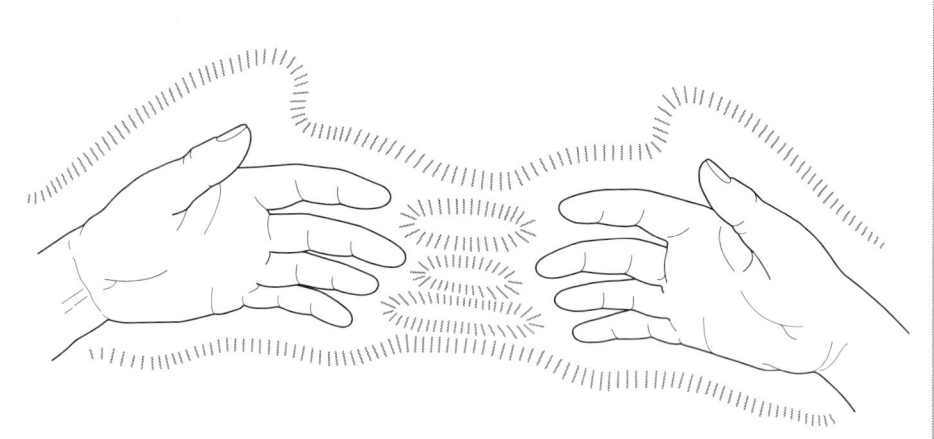

Figure 2. Sensing your hands' energies

If you can find an interested partner, get them to help you work with another pair of hands, as in this exercise.

EXERCISE 4

Sensing the energies of a partner's hands

- Stand opposite your partner at a distance where you can just touch each other's palms when your arms are fully extended. Both of you hold your palms up at about chest height, with the elbows bent, to face your partner's palms. Let the hands relax so that the fingers separate naturally.

- Slowly move your right palm to meet your partner's left palm. Then move your left palm to meet your partner's right palm.

exercise continues ▶

Gently pull your palms backwards towards you. Let your partner try these same movements. These are the same kind of movements you tried in the previous exercise.

- Now both of you move both sets of palms together. Slowly pull them back again. Notice what you sense. Was it different from sensing your own energies? Discuss the sensations with your partner.

Your hands are receptive to energies, as you have experienced. Let's see what happens when you encourage this process with visualisation.

EXERCISE 5
Breathing energy into the hands

- Sit comfortably with your feet flat on the ground. Rest your hands on your thighs, palms up (there is an energy centre in your palm which is receptive to subtle energies. By keeping your palms up you are in receptive mode). Breathe normally. Relax your elbows, the back of your neck and the tops of your shoulders. Do this by 'letting go' with each out-breath. Close your eyes if this helps you to concentrate.

- Focus on the centre of your palms. Visualise energy as light beaming down into them. Note what you feel or sense.

- Now visualise that you can 'breathe' this energy *into* your palms. As you see the energy beaming down, breathe in. On the in-breath, the energy is absorbed into your hands. On the out-breath, it fills your hands and arms.

exercise continues ▶

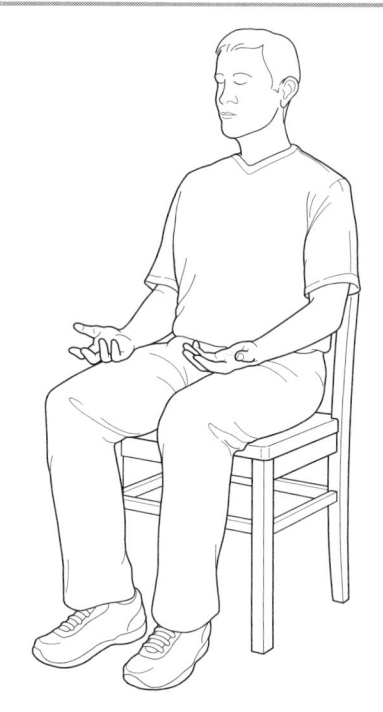

Figure 3. Breathing energy into the hands

Note your sensations and compare with the first part of the exercise. Follow this with the next exercise.

EXERCISE 6

Sending out energy from your hands

- Still sitting in the same position, raise your hands to about chest height with the palms facing away from the body.

- Visualise that you can beam energy *out* from your palms. What do you sense?

- Fill your hands with energy on the in-breath as you did in the previous exercise. Send out the energy on the out-breath.

exercise continues ▶

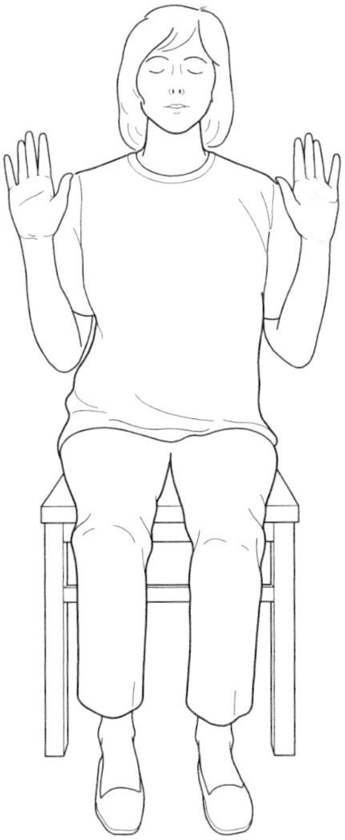

Figure 4. Sending out energy from the hands

Now try with a partner.

EXERCISE 7
Sending energy to a partner

- Sit opposite your partner, who should be sitting at least 2m (6ft) away from you. Both of you hold your hands up to about chest height, with the elbows bent, and the palms facing towards each other's. Your partner remains receptive. Take three full breaths into the abdomen to energise yourself. Breathe in. On the out-breath send energy from your hands to the palms of your partner's hands. Repeat.

- Now try beaming energy to your partner's hands by thought alone. Note all your sensations.

exercise continues ▶

> Change roles, with your partner carrying out each stage of the exercise. Again, note your sensations. What did receiving energy from your partner feel like? Compare notes together.

Experiencing subtle energies – the early stages

You are beginning to experience what happens to your hands when they are in contact with subtle energy, for example, a tingling sensation or heat. This is what might happen when you are ready to work. One of the signals that your work is complete may be the cessation of tingling or heat. Make a note of the signals that your hands give – they will be personal to you and they may be your own signal that you are ready to begin.

These sensations show that you have begun to experience subtle energies and some of the subtle aspects of your own, and perhaps your partner's, body. The following chapter provides you with the next essential step in understanding and appreciating your 'light' body.

Chapter 3

Your light body

Our work will bring us into contact with many aspects of human life, and perhaps other life forms as well. It will be quite natural to find ourselves pondering: Who am I? Where did I come from and what really is a body?

Let's look more closely, then, at the person we think we are.

The body is a spiritual creation

The Distant Healer acknowledges that Earth exists as a unique destination for the journeying soul and needs to be honoured and celebrated as such. Each of us, when we come to Earth, embarks on a life adventure that will be unique to us. We do not know where anyone else is on their soul journey. We do not know why people or situations present themselves as they do. What we do know is that, when we send out Distant Healing, for a time we are journeying together. For these reasons our work is always unconditional.

Soul, or our Higher Self, first has contact with creation through an energy pattern that can be envisaged as a 'body' of light. This light is vibrating at a frequency far beyond the speed of physical light and is another term for 'spirit' – the energy of the Source. But to engage in the total experience of physicality, soul needs the much denser energy form of the physical body. Then, to be conscious of this state, we also have the mental abilities of mind: the capability to create thought; intelligence:

which determines the level and quality of thought; and will: the power to drive thought into action. Mental energies travel at a far greater speed, and vibrate at a far greater frequency, than the body and so project beyond it, creating an energy 'body' invisible to normal sight but detectable by our subtle senses. All thoughts, their actions, interactions and reactions are processed in this mental body.

When thoughts interact with physical life, emotions are generated by the individual personality. These emotional energies, though not vibrating as fast as thought, still vibrate at a far greater rate than the physical body and so, again, project beyond it, creating another energy 'body'. Here, our emotions and emotional reactions are processed. Feelings generated by the Higher Self, to act as signals of warning, confirmation or guidance, are also processed in this 'emotional' part of our being.

Thus our spiritual, mental and emotional levels, or bodies, all vibrate at speeds greater than the speed of light. Their energies are *subtle*. As you have already found, they can be detected by us through the subtle senses. This is also true of other beings, such as animals – you may have noticed this with a pet. We all have this natural ability, which is actually essential to our survival. If you were not already aware of it, you will find that practising Distant Healing is a good way to reactivate it.

Because of the vast differences between the vibratory frequencies of the body and the frequencies of our spiritual, mental and emotional levels, there is an energetic bridging level known as the *etheric*. The etheric is also a subtle level, but its energies travel at speeds only just above the speed of light. Here, greater frequencies are stepped down in order to be made more compatible with the body energies.

For Distant Healers, the physical body with its symptoms is usually the presenting problem. But you may also be asked to help people with emotional, mental or even spiritual issues, all of which originate at one of the subtle levels described, in one or more of the subtle bodies.

The human energy field

I have described us as spiritual beings with an energy pattern designed for manifesting and experiencing life at the physical level – here on planet Earth and the rest of the universe. Because of its various energies, this energy pattern appears as a *series* of energy bodies. This may give the impression that, energetically, we are something like a set of Russian dolls, of bodies within bodies. The important difference is that the different rates of vibration allow the various bodies to be interpenetrating rather than simply one inside the other.

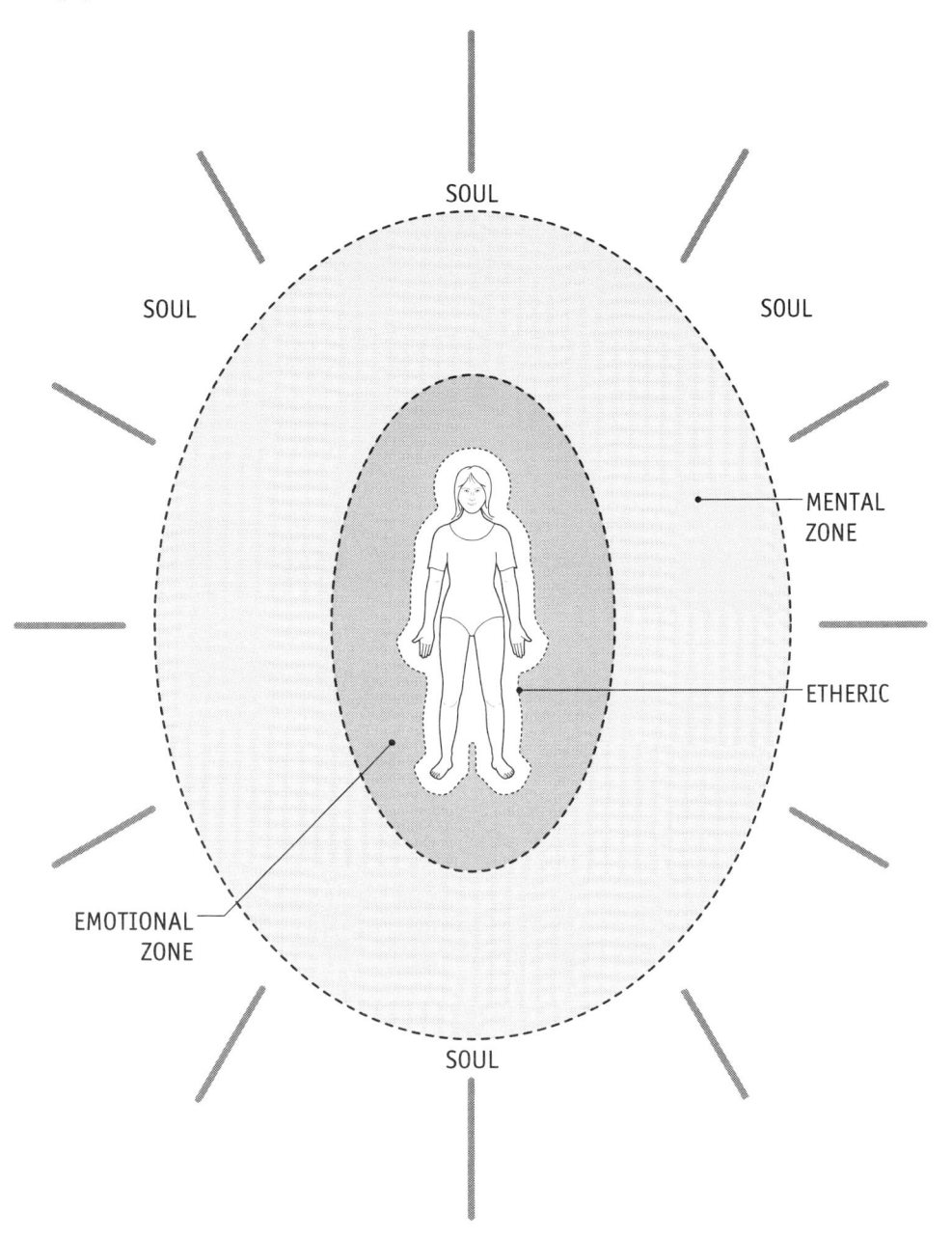

Figure 5. The human energy field

In other words, the soul part of you is right here, where 'you' are. So are the mental, emotional and etheric parts of you. In reality they are one, aspects of the whole you. Each body radiates its specific energies, creating a total field around us, known to the Ancient Greeks as the *aura*. To subtle sensing this appears as a glowing emanation which some people sense as different moving colours, while others may be aware of the field as sound, feelings, indescribable sensations, or personal information, such as a recent experience.

Encountering another energy field

When we encounter another person, we tend to decide very quickly if we like them or not, or whether they will be good for us or not. This is because at a subtle level we immediately sense their energy field and this gives us instant information about them. The relative energies of our fields are the basis of compatibility. Of course our mind can, and often does, override our intuition or subtle sensing. Perhaps the subtle information is negative, but they actually *look* nice to us. We can choose whether to listen to the message from our intuition or our mind. These factors apply to situations too.

All situations have an energy field and we can be aware of the information in the field or not, and take appropriate action or not. When we are asked for help as Distant Healers, we are presented with a person within a situation. Since we try to work unconditionally, we may wish to accept each case as it comes. But this does not prevent us from acting on an inner prompting not to accept a certain case. There may be a reason for this which will unfold later.

Let's make some practical discoveries about energy fields. You will need a partner for the next exercise.

EXERCISE 8

Sensing the energy field

- First, see if you can locate the edge or boundary of your partner's field. Your partner should stand in a relaxed position and breathe

exercise continues ▶

normally without focusing on what you are doing. Stand a good ten paces away from your partner. Relax by letting go of any tensions on the out-breath. Take as long as you need.

- Hold your hands up in front of you with the arms bent and the palms facing your partner. Put your attention into your previously activated palms (see Exercise 2: Activating the palm centres, page 21).

- Now walk very slowly towards your partner and stop as soon as you feel a slight energetic resistance, as if making contact with the surface of an invisible balloon. You are sensing the 'edge' of your partner's energy field. Move your hands over and around the invisible surface so that you get a picture of its shape. Note the shape that you have actually defined (see Figure 6 below). Step back from your partner and relax.

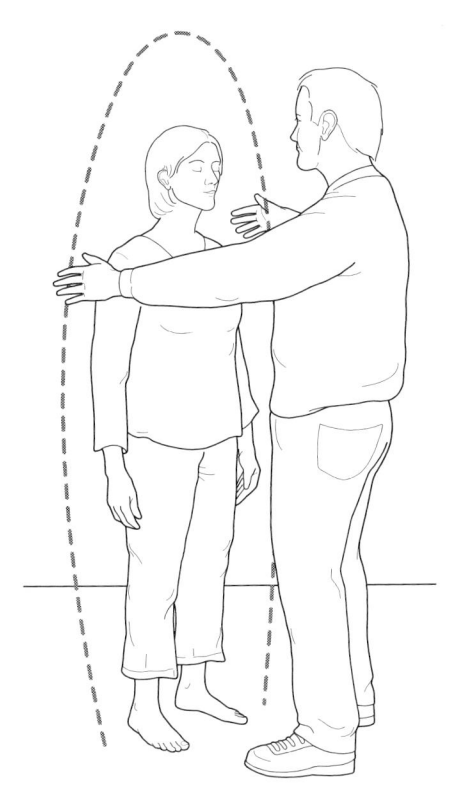

Figure 6. Sensing the energy field

exercise continues ▶

- Hold up your hands again, facing your partner. Now see if you can sense another 'layer' of energy in your partner's field as you move very slowly towards him or her. The more relaxed you are, the easier it will be to sense the denser layers of the field as you move nearer to your partner's body.

- Finally, decide how many zones of energy you were able to sense in your partner's field, where they seemed to be located and what shape they seemed to have.

- Change roles to let your partner work with you. Compare experiences.

The next exercise introduces you to the information stored as various energies in the energy field. Again, you will need to work with a partner. The exercise should last from two to five minutes.

EXERCISE 9

Sensing information in the energy field

- Sit opposite each other without being close enough to touch. Both of you relax and breathe normally. Your partner should be as passive as possible. Both of you close your eyes to avoid absorbing visual information.

- As you sit opposite your partner, realise that their energy field includes mental and emotional material. Allow yourself to be open to this material and see if you become aware of it.

- Visualise that your whole body is open to this energetic material. What are you aware of? Make a mental note of it, no matter how strange or ordinary it may seem.

- Relax for a few minutes and change roles.

- Finally, share and compare notes together.

This last exercise may require practice before you are able to sense material in a partner's field. Although you need to be relaxed, you also need to be totally aware. When we come to certain forms of distant healing later in the book, you will find that this exercise has been particularly useful in preparing you for them.

The etheric body

Healing energies make contact with a person at the etheric bridging level. In practice the etheric body can be seen as a misty layer of light, projecting 2–5cm (1–2in) or so beyond the physical body, most often visible to normal vision when a person is standing against a white or pale background. It extends beyond the body because its energies are vibrating at a slightly faster rate. The etheric body has a shape somewhat like the human form, with an outer surface composed of a glowing web-like structure, the whole appearing to be illuminated from within.

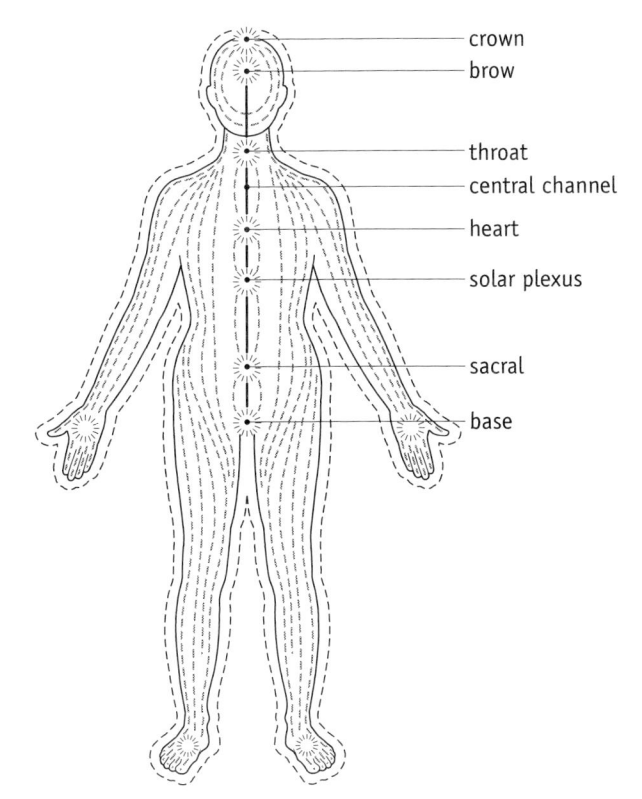

Figure 7. The etheric body and the seven main energy centres

The luminous depths are seen to contain hundreds of even brighter lines of light. These transparent channels permit the flow of a range of subtle energies which appear as moving streams or threads of light. Where the channels intersect, a node or vortex of light is formed. The effect is to give the etheric body the appearance of a starry sky at night. Many of these etheric channels correspond to the meridians used in acupuncture.

The nodes of light are the subtle energy centres of the etheric body (see also *chakra* in the Glossary, page 193*)*. The more channels that converge, the larger the energy centre and the more prominent are its activities. All centres are engaged in some aspect of processing and monitoring of energy flow. The seven main centres are seen to be connected to a central channel aligned with the spine (see Figure 7 on the previous page). Their function is to allow the flow of energy to and from the various levels of our being and to process the energies generated by specific life issues. Because their roles are crucial to human life, and therefore to Distant Healing, we will study them in more detail in Part Two.

Armed with the essential knowledge about your body and its subtle, or 'light', aspects you almost have what you need to make a start with Distant Healing. Before you do that, however, I want to make sure that you begin with the best possible grounding and that you are properly equipped for your healing 'journey' from the outset. These preparations, which you will need from now on, are essential.

Chapter 4

Preparations for getting started

Taking up the challenge

When we make the choice to act (instead of doing nothing), and to send positive energies out to someone or some situation (instead of a negative thought), we take up the challenge to remember Oneness, and the essential nature of our being: Love.

Our action has to be as natural, spontaneous and unconditional as any other loving or compassionate gesture. This is a step on the way to self-empowerment, yes, but if you find yourself doing it, you can be sure that you have the Distant Healing attitude. It is an attitude that ensures that you will have the motivation, and the energy, to enjoy practising Distant Healing.

The work is a two-way process involving many responsibilities: to oneself as well as to the person we are working with. Even though the person may never know we are sending out to them, we need to bear in mind that we have entered into the sacred relationship of Distant Healing where both parties are equal. The reality of the other person becomes our reality, and the energetic flow will affect us too.

As I indicated earlier, healing energies work simultaneously at the spiritual, mental and emotional levels, as well as with the physical body. They will tend to go where there is the greatest need so effects may not necessarily show up on the physical. This may mean some of the people we are working with find themselves needing to reassess their lives, looking at what is most important and what their priorities should be; what causes distress and what can be done about those causes; understanding the effects of thoughts and emotions and how much they are in control of them. However, these impacts only occur because of synchronicity – at the time a person is ready and able to deal with them. We can be assured, too, that the process is gentle and loving.

Beginning the process of attunement

We can now expand our initial choice to take positive and caring action by some conscious preparation. Much of the energy radiated by us humans has been generated by thought and is of a relatively heavy nature. Some of this is in the universal energy field around us; some we absorb from other people; and some is transmitted to us via thought. Knowing that we are surrounded by, and absorb, the energies of life – the buildings and objects, situations and people whom we encounter – we first prepare ourselves to work as Distant Healers by clearing, balancing and energising our own energy field. This is the total field of energy that we all generate from the different levels of our being, which changes as our life experience changes, moment by moment. Because the Distant Healing process takes place within the energy field, we will look at it again in Part Two.

Clearing, balancing and energising our own energy field begins the process of attunement to the Source of healing energies. As you found in the first exercise, attunement is aligning your individual self with the Higher Self and the subtle energies. Your level of attunement will determine the quality and quantity of the energy you initiate and channel. The exercises in this chapter will raise your level of attunement and deepen your experience of Exercise 1, on page 17. Your approach to them should be enthusiastic, but totally relaxed. There are no deadlines and healing is never about competition.

The benefits of effective posture

I mentioned how breathing is the key to energising ourselves; and how breathing is influenced by our posture. The effective standing posture has the same energising aim – a relaxed body and a relaxed mind, where you can pay attention while letting all thoughts pass through your mind unobstructed. You will be able to practise this in the next exercise, which removes any energy that might impede your attunement. The exercise uses the clearing energy of silver light. The standing stance described opens up the field and allows energy to flow freely.

EXERCISE 10
Clearing the energy field

- Stand, or sit if necessary, with your feet a shoulder-width apart, your arms hanging loosely by your sides. Gently flex the knees and allow your body to relax. Use the breath to help relaxation and attunement.

- As you become aware that your centre of gravity is just below the navel, breathe in the same way as before, gently into the abdomen. Enjoy the feeling of being relaxed, yet alert. This is the state to aim for whenever an exercise calls for a standing posture.

- Take a moment to be aware of any heavy energy in your body and energy field, noting where it seems to have accumulated. (It is worth making a note of this observation in your journal, every time you do this exercise, to see if there is a pattern.)

- Now visualise yourself under a shower or gentle waterfall of silver light. Let this light pour over you, through you and out into your surrounding field, especially to any place where you sensed an accumulation of heavy energy. Allow the light to exit through your hands and feet and every body orifice.

- Notice the colour of the light that moves in to fill the space that you have cleared. Your awareness of this will confirm that the clearing is taking place. Remember, you could sense this in a number of ways. If you feel you are sensing nothing (it is your mind saying you can't), carry out this important exercise as if you can.

- Note the sensations of clearing and the sensations of being cleansed.

exercise continues ▶

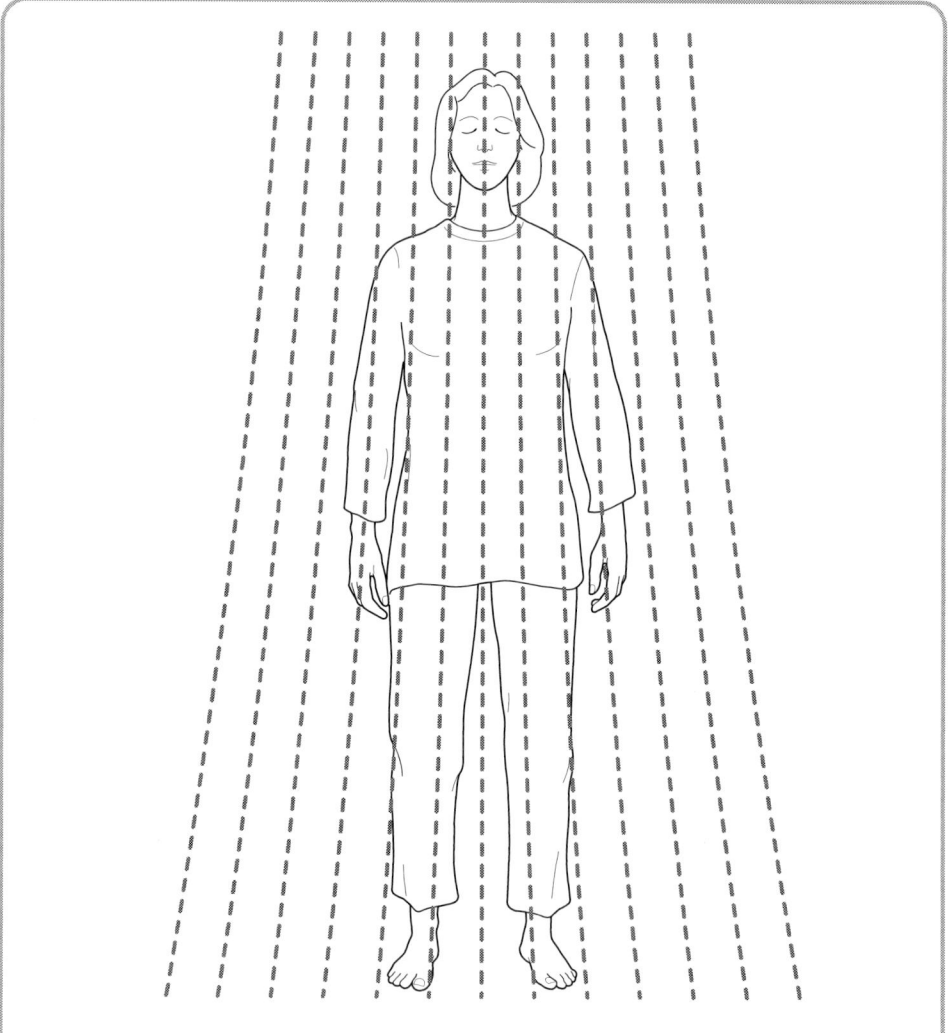

Figure 8. Clearing the energy field

- Continue to breathe naturally and take a few moments to be with these sensations.

Now you are ready to bring balance and stability to your energy field with the next exercise.

EXERCISE 11

The Rainbow Breath

Note: Anyone experiencing breathing difficulties should only attempt the exercises involving conscious breathing under supervision.

Before practising this exercise, refresh your picture of the seven main energy centres (chakras). When in a state of balance they each vibrate to one of the rainbow colours, ranging from the base to the crown (see Figure 7, page 33).

- Stand, or sit if necessary, with your feet a shoulder-width apart, with your arms hanging loosely by your sides. Relax your body.

- Take three or more breaths to clear the lungs. Allow any tension, worry or anxieties to exit as you exhale through your open mouth. Close your mouth and breathe normally when you feel settled.

- You are now going to fill your energy field with seven spheres of coloured light, ranging from red to violet. Each sphere should be visualised as outside the one you created before.

- Breathe in, visualising red light rising from behind your heels, moving up your back to the top of your head. Pause for a moment.

- As you exhale, visualise the red light also spreading down the front of your body until it is under your feet. You are now enclosed in a sphere of red light and ready to build your personal energy rainbow.

- Breathe up a sphere of orange light, spreading it in the same way by using the breath, making sure it totally encloses the sphere of red light.

- Breathe up golden yellow light and surround the orange light sphere.

- Breathe up green light and surround the golden yellow light sphere.

exercise continues ▶

- Breathe up sky-blue light and surround the green light sphere.
- Breathe up royal-blue/indigo light and surround the sky blue light sphere.
- Breathe up violet/purple light and surround the royal blue/indigo light sphere.
- Spend a few moments of awareness as you are totally enclosed in the seven spheres of rainbow light. They are, of course, aspects of the one white light, but by working with them separately you are able to balance the seven main energy centres of your subtle energy body.

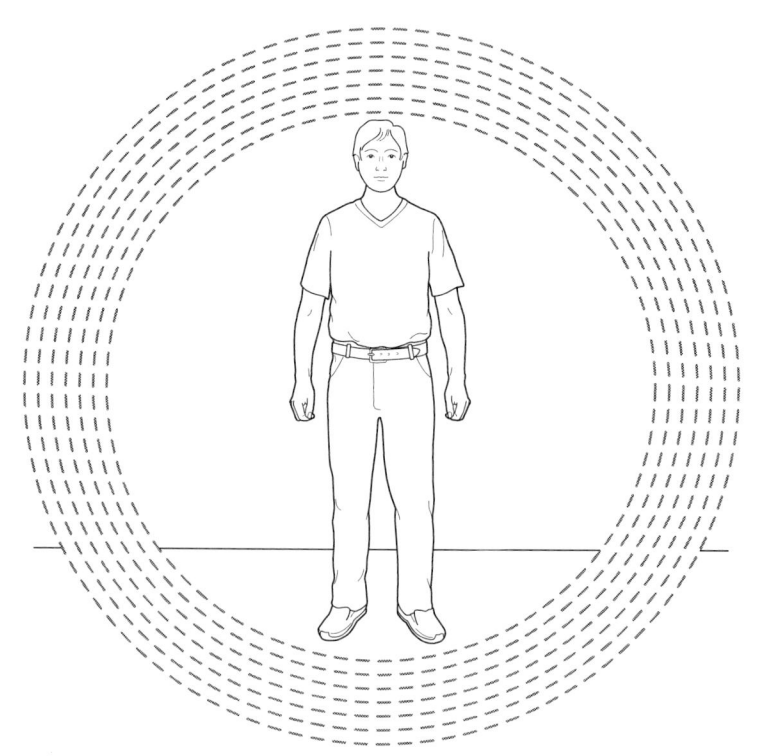

Figure 9. The Rainbow Breath

Pausing to be with the effects of this exercise can put you in touch with deep parts of yourself. What do you experience: a sense of peace, of balance, of healing? This is you.

The breath and breathing

This brings us to the role of breathing in your life and in your work as a Distant Healer. Although all of us begin breathing from the moment of birth, and we know that our life depends on it, most people do not know how to breathe properly; neither do they know about the spiritual dimension of their own breath.

This second aspect of the sacred breath will gradually become apparent as you practise the exercises, most of which use the breath to ease tension, bring balance, calm and relaxation, and facilitate the attunement process. This opens the way for the beneficial presence and influence of the Higher Self. Part of the life skill of Distant Healing is the gift of conscious breathing.

How breathing works

The action of the large muscle forming the floor of the chest, the diaphragm, is what allows us to breathe. When the diaphragm is flattened downwards, the cavity enclosed by the rib cage is enlarged, creating a vacuum. The lungs are suspended in this cavity and they immediately expand to fill the space, drawing in air via the nose or mouth. Once the lungs are full, a nervous impulse signals the diaphragm to relax upwards. This deflates the lungs, forcing the breath to be expelled.

As air is breathed into the lungs, oxygen passes through their fine membranes into the bloodstream to oxygenate the cells and tissues of the whole body. Waste gases from the bodily processes, such as carbon dioxide, leave the bloodstream via the lungs to be expelled.

There are thus two breaths, the in-breath and the out-breath, each of which has a different sensation and a specific purpose. It is interesting to note that the first thing we do at birth is take an in-breath: we engage with the receptive, or 'feminine', energy stream. This is reversed at the death of the body with the final emissive act of the 'masculine' energy stream: the out-breath. These two breaths mark the beginning and end of the sacred breathing cycle which is vital to life.

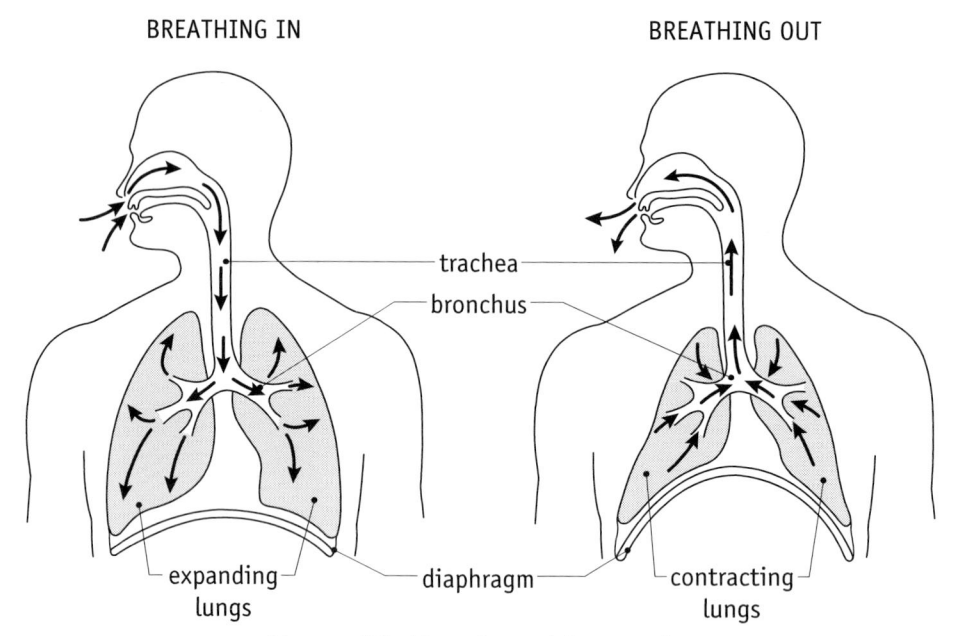

Figure 10. How breathing works

The effects of disturbed breathing

Unless we suffer from a respiratory disorder, we tend not to think about breathing. It is automatic, under the control of the autonomic nervous system. Like the other systems of the body, we do not have to send a message to our breathing apparatus to keep going since it is a function of the co-ordinated living body. However, in any group of people there are breathing habits that range from the highly efficient to the dangerously inefficient; the latter having long-term implications for health.

When we are upset, our breathing rate and heartbeat increase due to the secretion of adrenaline. By controlling our breathing and calming it, we can regain the balance of mind and emotions. This sends a message to the adrenal glands to stop secreting adrenaline so that breathing and heartbeat are further calmed.

Disturbed breathing also affects the proper movement of the diaphragm. This is inhibited so that it upsets normal breathing rhythm, but it can be remedied by the simple act of controlling our breathing.

The subtle role of breathing

The cycle of the breath is the basic, physical function of breathing. But it also carries the subtle life force (Sanskrit *prana*, Chinese *qi*), to every part of the body via the blood system. This ability of the breath to carry subtle energies means that we are able to take in healing energies from the energy field and through conscious breathing.

The breath of life is so much more than our unconscious breathing in and out. When the newborn baby takes its first breath it is an affirmation of the role of air as the carrier of oxygen and the life force. Just as the in-breath is a way of taking in, and receiving, what we need, so the out-breath is a signal for energy to escape. Anything that needs to escape, to be released or to find a way out of the system, can do so with the out-breath. When you use the breath in this way, to let go of stress or anxiety for example, it is helpful to do it with an open mouth since this reminds you that your conscious out-breath has this function.

The next exercise will introduce you to the benefits of breathing more fully and deeply. If you have any form of breathing difficulty, please take note of the following proviso: *all exercises in this book that involve conscious breathing should only be carried out under supervision.*

EXERCISE 12

Full-breath breathing

This exercise re-educates your physical body to return to efficient energy breathing, maximising available energies for intake and output. It rebalances the whole system and realigns all aspects of your being.

- Sit comfortably with your feet flat on the ground. Notice your breathing. Allow it to become slow, deep and gentle.

- Notice what your chest and abdomen are doing. In full-breath breathing, the focus is on the movement of the abdomen, rather

exercise continues ▶

than the chest. Put your hands there and imagine it is a balloon you are going to fill and then empty.

- As you slowly inhale through the nose, allow your 'balloon' to fill by letting your abdomen gently expand. Do not strain.

- Exhale slowly and feel the balloon of your abdomen deflate. Again, do not strain.

- Practise this exercise three times. Note the difference between the in-breath and the out-breath. Note how you feel as you breathe like this.

The next time you see a sleeping baby, notice the way the baby breathes. How different is this to the way you generally breathe? Full-breath breathing is also known as 'soft-belly' breathing because it encourages the relaxation of the abdomen and discourages the tense, hard-belly approach to body posture. Breathing and posture affect our mood and attitude. They can easily be trained to affect both in a positive way. The soft-belly posture allows you to breathe deeply and gently so that you are calm and balanced, with your centre of gravity below your navel.

Full-breath breathing may also be used as a self-healing activity to improve breathing capacity and rhythm, to benefit the whole physical system.

Relaxation

The next attunement step of conscious relaxation goes hand in hand with conscious breathing. Relaxation relieves tension and stress at all levels, allowing the body energies to flow more freely. The activities of the brain, heart and lungs are slowed down, calming the mind and emotions. This creates the ideal state for attunement, Distant Healing and meditation.

The following exercise is a simple, yet thorough method of relaxing the whole body. In it you send a command to the brain to allow all the muscles to relax, release and let go. You co-ordinate this with slow, deep and gentle breathing, which immediately sends positive messages to all the body systems that things are becoming calm and peaceful. Once your body and mind are acquainted with the feeling of relaxation, you will be able to move into relaxation mode at will. This will be an essential element in your attunement procedure.

EXERCISE 13

Full-body relaxation

You may find it useful to record the exercise or have it read out to you by your working partner.

- Ideally, you should lie on a firm, even surface with a comfortable support for your head and neck.

- Allow your legs to part slightly and move your hands away from the sides of your body. Carry out the full breath three times as in the previous exercise. Breathe slowly, gently and normally.

- Now focus on your hands. Clench them tightly to make a fist and let them unclench with the out-breath. Remember the feeling of unclenching (relaxing) and letting go as you exhale. Do not clench anything again throughout the rest of this exercise. As you breathe, know that you are breathing in peace and relaxation. Let any anxieties or problems go with the out-breath and breathe them out through the open mouth.

- Bring your focus to the toes of your left foot. Feel them relax, one by one. Use the out-breath to let go, release and relax. Move slowly over your foot, relaxing the muscles. Let the ankle go.

- Move up your left leg, relaxing the muscles. Let the knee joint go. Relax the thigh muscles and the muscles of the buttocks.

- Let go across the pelvis. Continue to breathe slowly and gently.

exercise continues ▶

- Focus on your right foot and proceed in the same way. Feel the toes relax, one by one. Move slowly over your right foot, relaxing the muscles, relaxing, letting go. Let the ankle go.

- Move up your right leg, let the knee joint go. Relax the thigh muscles and the muscles of the buttocks. Relax the pelvis again.

- Now move your attention up the front of your body, relaxing the belly and stomach. Let go of the muscles of the chest. Let go of the shoulders.

- Return your attention to the lower back and slowly relax your back muscles, one by one. Remember to use the out-breath to let go and unclench. Make sure you take the time to relax them all if you suffer from back pain. Pay attention to the muscles across the top of your back and shoulders where tension tends to gather. Relax and let go.

- Relax the left shoulder and move down the left arm. Let the elbow joint go. Move down the forearm, relaxing and letting go. Let the wrist relax.

- Relax the palm, thumb and fingers, one by one.

- Return to the right shoulder. Relax it and move down the right arm. Let the elbow joint go. Move down the forearm, relaxing and letting go. Let the wrist relax.

- Relax the right hand, letting go of your thumb and fingers one by one. Relax the whole shoulder girdle.

- Now move up the back of your neck, very slowly, relaxing and letting go. Let your attention come up the back of your head and over the top of the scalp, relaxing and letting go of all the tiny muscles.

- Imagine a caring hand smoothing your forehead. Relax the eyes, the cheeks, the mouth, the jaw.

- Continue to breathe slowly, gently and normally. Scan your body to see if any part has tensed up again. If it has, relax it, enjoying the

exercise continues ▶

> feeling of total relaxation. At this point you can remain mentally alert or allow yourself to drift off into sleep.
>
> When you repeat this exercise, try starting the relaxation at the top of your body, making your way down to the toes, using the same technique. See which order is most comfortable for you. You may find that you need to use a different order to suit different times or circumstances. Practise relaxation so that it becomes second nature and you can do it anywhere, in any circumstance, in any position. This exercise facilitates a loving communication with every aspect of your physical form, re-establishing a positive relationship with the body.

Addressing your work space

Distant Healing can be carried out anywhere and at any time, but you will probably carry out most of your practice indoors, perhaps in a space dedicated to this. Use the following guidance on attuning your work space according to where you wish to practise.

Your work space has an energy field, no matter what its location or size. Just as you need to be attuned to the Source, so does the space. First, pay attention to its physical aspects. It should be clean and fresh. Next, clear, balance and harmonise the room or space, as you did with yourself. This can be done with smoke, such as incense. It is the same technique as the Native American 'smudging' with sage or some other herb. The smoke is wafted into all areas of the room. Some healers like to use a light source, such as a candle; or a sound source, such as a bell or the clapping of hands. You can even visualise your work space being cleared and balanced in the same way that you worked on yourself with colour. What colour of energy does your room need to be filled with? Make a note and see if this colour changes the next time you need to work there. Perhaps you have a special ritual, prayers, chants or songs. This is fine. Your intention guides the process. The next exercise, using an incense stick, is a suggestion along these lines that you can adapt in any way you wish. Note what the various actions are for.

EXERCISE 14

Preparing and dedicating the work space

Use some of the earlier procedures to calm and relax. Finally, put your mind in your heart centre (in the middle of your chest). Take a few moments to breathe in and out of this centre. Light an incense stick. Dedicate the light and smoke to the Light of healing. Ask for protection as you open yourself to be a channel for healing energies. Ask for help to be as pure a channel as possible.

- Ask that the smoke may be used to clear, balance and harmonise your space.

- Remain focused as you hold the incense stick and intuitively face a certain direction of the space. Move in a circle from where you are standing, allowing the smoke to spread out into the space before you. Take your time and do not hurry this procedure. Use your other hand to help waft the smoke over the furniture, especially any chairs, and into any corners.

- If you find that you need to move in an anticlockwise direction, you are clearing the energies of the space. If you find that you need to move in a sunwise (clockwise) direction, you are filling the space with new energies and raising the energy level.

- As you move round you might like to ask that the space be cleared of all energies that are not compatible with healing. Ask that the space be filled with the energies of healing: the energies of Peace, Love and Light. Ask for a blessing on the space and all who enter it, or give a blessing yourself.

- If you work in a building shared by others, ask for a blessing on the room, the building and all who work (and live) in it.

- Wait for an intuitive signal that the job of clearing and dedicating the space has been completed.

There is plenty of scope here for your own favourite methods, but check intuitively if they feel right for the task of Distant Healing which is to follow. Any room or space, whether inside or outside, is conscious, but attunement raises this consciousness by accelerating the vibrations of the field, just as it raises the vibrations of your own energy field.

Much of the energetic activity of attunement occurs on a subtle level, involving energies that vibrate faster than the speed of light. Recall that you have a subtle energy system designed to process these energies, the energies of healing and the other subtle energies that are vital to our lives as physical, emotional, mental and spiritual beings.

Attunement to the source of healing energies

Having attuned your Distant Healing space, you can move to the final step in your own attunement. Attunement is very much based on your conscious intention and you may well find that your work on the space has brought you to a place of total quiet focus, especially if you have carried it out with your mind focused on your heart centre. Now practise Exercise 1: Attunement, page 17, again to compare your deeper sense of attunement with your initial experience in Chapter 1.

Remember that attunement, with your focus in the heart centre, is the key element in all your Distant Healing work. If you wish to use it as a form of meditation, practise in the morning and evening. Start with a few minutes each session, gently building it up to half an hour over a period of weeks.

Having set up the first side of that powerful energetic structure – the Healing Triangle – you are now ready to work.

Positive attitudes mean good preparation

Distant Healing can be applied to people, animals, plants, a landscape and also to situations. From a healing point of view, situations have moved to the top of the list in terms of priority. This does not mean that individuals no longer matter, far from it. But we are all living in a time when the situations and circumstances in which individuals find themselves range through the dangerous, tragic, painful, extremely stressful, confrontational and life threatening – to name but some of them. Our time calls for new forms of action and commitment. When people feel disempowered, and under threat, they become victims of fear. Some fear turns to violent and destructive action, some to apathy and cynicism. The life situations that daily appear on our screens and radios, and in our news media, are the giant wounds that need urgent healing. Those 'on the ground', facing up to or living with these wounds, need more help than they will ever physically get.

This is where Distant Healing comes in. I told you the story about the young pregnant woman and her situation to illustrate how healing energies address the whole energetic situation that surrounds someone. Not only were the young woman and her baby helped, but the behaviour and mind-sets of others in her life were altered for the better. Now imagine these possibilities enlarged to whatever scale they may be vitally needed.

From now on, every time you are confronted with some fearful vision or other, or some dreadful news, realise that you are far from powerless to do something. But positive thinking alone is not enough. Positive thinking may help *you* to cope, but it won't make much difference to the violence or suffering that is going on at some distance from you. Because of Oneness, in some way it is happening to all of us too.

There is a biblical story about the first humans, Eve and Adam. They were having fun discovering the abundance of the primeval Garden when the Holy One called out: 'Where are you?' This is often taken to mean that Eve and Adam were hiding – as if the One who made everything, including them and the Garden, did not know where they were! Another level of meaning, taught by New Mexico rabbi, Gershon Winkler, is that the Holy One was actually asking them: 'Where are *you*? Where is your *consciousness now* – is it confined to awareness of your wonderful bodies and the physical world around you, or is it also aligned with Oneness?' This deeper meaning is a good reminder about where we need to be whenever we contemplate Distant Healing.

Now fully prepared, in the next chapter we will make a start as Distant Healers. Later, we will also look at the benefits of sharing the work with others, in the form of a Distant Healing group.

Chapter 5

Baseline practice

Creating a Healing list

We begin with the fundamental practice of Distant Healing that you will be able to adapt to the various calls that come your way. You will need to start a Distant Healing Book. In this you make a note of all the persons, animals, landscapes, situations etc. that you are going to send out to. This is your Distant Healing list. If someone has been referred to you, make a note of the date and ask the referrer to keep in touch and let you know at regular intervals how the person concerned is getting on.

The name has a vibration which is an important energetic link with you, and so with the healing forces involved. When working with something like a landscape or a situation, note when you begin work and do your own monitoring. You may also like to compile a 'scrapbook' of relevant press cuttings of events, situations and other illustrated material. Gradually, your Distant Healing Book begins to reveal the pattern of your work.

Your preparations foster at-onement and a positive mindset. The positive mindset is to be happy in your work, to look forward to it, while not being attached to outcome. Distant Healing is a way of developing and practising unconditional love: the true gift of the heart. This unconditional attitude implies non-attachment, but total empathy with the subject and those who may be asking for your help. Distant Healing encourages you to approach the work so that each case has your unconditional positive regard and each case is of equal value.

The energetic law of attraction means that, once you have indicated to the Source that you are available to work, people will seek your help and situations will present themselves. This happens when the time is right for your paths to cross and it is especially true in the case of a person or an animal. The moment of meeting has been arranged at a soul level with the agreement of all concerned. It is a moment of sacred synchronicity. A telephone call from the patient is particularly effective because it carries the vibration of the caller to you. This will be activated later when you come across their name, or the name of the third party, on your list.

How the subject can help

When people ask for your help, either for themselves or a third party, asking them to give you a progress report encourages them to take responsibility for their requests. Patients can then be further empowered by your asking them to help you by joining in. Ideally, this is at the same time as the healing is being sent, but it is not crucial. (As explained earlier, the energies travel outside of the space-time continuum.) Invite patients to sit or lie quietly at the time you will be sending out to them. Ask them to relax, breathe normally and visualise a sphere of protective light around them. They should remain like this for 15 minutes if possible.

When subjects are able to join you in this way, they frequently sense the energies in all kinds of ways and are able to give you feedback about their experience. This may or may not coincide with your experience of their healing. It is always interesting and a way of demonstrating the many wonderful ways in which healing energy manifests.

The unconditional intention

Because energy follows thought, it travels at the level of that thought. This energy law means that the Distant Healer should pay attention to the way the request for help is made, taking care to avoid being influenced by this. For example, the requester tells you that they have a friend who has been diagnosed with bronchitis which was caused by smoking. 'You should send some extra healing in case he develops lung cancer, and he probably needs help to give up his addiction to nicotine as well.'

In such cases, you will need to listen dispassionately to the request without taking on board the statements and feelings around it. In your response, you take care to say that your way of working is to send healing to the person not the condition, without sounding as if you are making a judgement about the requester. All you need is the name of the subject and to know whether they have agreed to accept Distant Healing help. These precautions are necessary because the initial impulse of love (the urge to ask for help) has become distorted by the mind-based opinions of the requester.

When this happens, the energy, travelling at the level of such thoughts, may be unwanted, unnecessary, or ineffective. This is why the Distant Healer does not attempt to direct the healing to a certain aspect or level of a person, though this may well occur during the healing process. In the same way, the unconditional nature of the work means that it cannot involve any kind of judgement or moral attitude towards the requester or possible third party subject.

The two methods of baseline practice

Each time you go to work as a Distant Healer, have your list ready, itemising who and what you wish to send out to. Your list should not be so long that you get tired or lose focus. Start with six to ten cases and a session of around half an hour. Gradually build your list until you find the optimum number for a fully effective and comfortable session. A long list may mean more than one session a week. However long or short your list, it is part of Distant Healing to always include requests for peace, healing for the planet and the Earth Family – all the other beings that dwell here with us.

There are two methods of baseline practice. In the first: you attune, receive the Light, and send that healing energy out to the subject. In the second: you attune, receive the Light, and put that healing energy in front of you to form a 'pool' or 'column'. The subject is then immersed in the healing energy pool or column. Through practising both these methods you will be fully prepared to work both ways with a group and for the more advanced work in Part Two.

EXERCISE 15

Sending out the healing Light

- Make sure the phone is disconnected and that you will not be disturbed. Attune your work space and attune yourself as outlined in the previous chapters.

- You may wish to light a candle as a symbol of the Light of the Source. If so, dedicate it to the work, and any helpers you might have in the spiritual realms. Give thanks that you have been given the opportunity to send out healing Light.

- Bring your focus to your heart centre. As you inhale, visualise this centre filling with the Light. With the next breath, the Light fills your chest.

- As you look over your list, ask for the Light to be sent out to each subject as you mention them one by one. You can say aloud or in your mind: 'I ask for healing to be sent to (name).' Carefully work through your list like this. Take your time, pausing if necessary. This simply means that you are in tune with what is happening energetically.

- When you reach the end of your list, give thanks.

- Rest assured that all those on your list have received healing they need. Sit quietly with your experience.

- When you have completed your work, blow out the candle. This can be done by sending out the light of the candle. Pause for a moment and see if you intuitively feel where it needs to go. This is usually the first place that comes to mind and could be to a person, a strife-ridden place, an environment under threat, etc. As you blow out the candle, say: 'I send the Light out to –.'

- Once you have closed your session, you have handed over the list to higher powers. It is time to stop thinking about your cases.

BASELINE PRACTICE • 55

In the early stages of practice, alternate the first basic technique of sending out the Light (as on p. 54) with the second basic technique of creating the Light pool or circle. This follows next.

EXERCISE 16
Creating the Light pool

- Make sure the phone is disconnected and that you will not be disturbed. Attune your work space and attune yourself as outlined in the previous chapters.

- You may wish to light a candle as a symbol of the Light of the Source. If so dedicate it to the work, and any helpers you might have in the spiritual realms. Give thanks that you have been given the opportunity to help others through the Light of Distant Healing.

- Bring your focus to your heart centre. As you inhale, visualise this centre filling with Light. With the next breath, the Light fills your chest.

- Now see this Light extending from you to a place in front of you to make an energy pool or circle.

- As you look over your list, ask for those on it to be put in the Light, mentioning them one by one. You can say aloud or in your mind: 'I ask for healing for (name).' Carefully work through your list like this. Take your time, pausing if necessary. This simply means that you are in tune with what is happening energetically.

- When you reach the end of your list, give thanks.

- Visualise that all those on the list have been gathered into the Light pool or circle. Here, they will receive healing they need. Sit quietly with your experience.

- When you have completed your work, blow out the candle. This can be done by sending out the light of the candle. Pause for a

exercise continues ▶

> moment and see if you intuitively feel where it needs to go. This is usually the first place that comes to mind. As you blow out the candle, say: 'I send the Light out to –.'
>
> - Once you have closed your session, you have handed over the list to higher powers. It is time to stop thinking about your cases.

Baseline practice: The Closing-down Procedure

Your baseline practice is complete only when you have carried out the essential Closing-down Procedure described below.

If you wish to follow a session with some other spiritual practice, such as meditation, you are in the ideal state to do this. If not, realise that the work has opened your energy centres more than is needed for everyday functioning. In other words, you no longer need to be open to that level of energy flow. You now need to carry out the following Closing-down Procedure to realign your centres and protect your energy field. This is particularly necessary if you are going to mix with other people in any way, such as going to the supermarket – for you would otherwise be too open to those energies.

When your Distant Healing session is in the evening, the Closing-down Procedure also ensures sound sleep. 'Closing down' refers to a procedure which returns your subtle energy system to everyday functioning; it is linked to your closing your working sessions. It does not mean fully closing the energy centres or shutting down any of the body systems.

Carrying out the Closing-down Procedure after each session of work will eventually become second nature. You can also use it to return your subtle energy system to everyday functioning at other times too. Even a conversation or reading a book about spiritual matters can open your centres. But remember that the centres should never be forcibly closed.

During the day most people absorb a variety of energies from other people, from places they visit, and from the things they do. Sensitive people, like healers and other therapists, tend to absorb even more into their energy fields. Some of these energies are incompatible with your own and you sense them through feelings of heaviness, restlessness, even depression. Realise that they are not *your* feelings and take appropriate steps to deal with them.

The first closing-down exercise clears incompatible energies. This is the same as Exercise 10 in Chapter 4. I repeat it here so that you don't have to turn back.

EXERCISE 10
Clearing the energy field

Recall that this exercise uses the clearing energy of silver light. The standing stance described in the following two exercises has important beneficial effects. It aligns the centres, facilitates grounding and frees the energy circuits to flow appropriately.

- Stand, or sit if necessary, with your feet a shoulder-width apart, your arms hanging loosely by your sides. Flex the knees and allow your body to relax. Use the breath to help relaxation and attunement.

- Take a moment to be aware of any heavy energy in your body and energy field, noting where it seems to have accumulated. (It is worth making a note of this observation in your journal, every time you do this exercise, to see if there is a pattern.)

- Now visualise yourself under a shower or gentle waterfall of silver light. Let this light pour over you, through you and out into your surrounding field, especially to any place where you sensed an accumulation of heavy energy. Allow the light to exit through your hands and feet and every body orifice (Figure 8, page 38).

- Notice the colour of the light that moves in to fill the space that you have cleared. Your awareness of this will confirm that the clearing is taking place. Remember, you could sense this in a number of ways. If you feel you are sensing nothing (it is your mind saying you can't), carry out this important exercise as if you can.

- Note the sensations of clearing and the sensations of being cleansed.

Next, we bring the centres from being wide open back to everyday functioning. First check that you remember the location of each of the seven main centres and their colours. If necessary, refer to Figure 7, page 33.

EXERCISE 17

Regulating the energy centres

For the purpose of the exercise, visualise your centres as rather like flowers with petals that are able to close up, but not shut tightly. The exercise is carried out by visualising the 'flowers' of each centre gently closing up a little. Your intention is to bring them to everyday functioning. See the colours as light.

- Standing relaxed with knees gently flexed, as in the previous exercise, start at the crown centre, which has the colour violet. Visualise it closing up a little.

- Move your awareness to the brow centre – colour indigo/royal blue. Close it up a little.

- Move to the throat centre – colour sky-blue. Close it up a little.

- Move to the heart centre – colour green. Close it up a little.

- Move to the solar plexus centre – colour golden yellow. Close it up a little.

- Move to the sacral centre – colour orange. Close it up a little.

- Move to the base centre – colour glowing red. Close it up a little.

- Now notice the first colour that comes to mind. This is the colour of energy that will keep your system in place. Surround yourself with a sphere of this light.

This is also a grounding process. Note the direction of activity: from the highest vibration of the crown centre to that closest to the Earth at the base centre.

The final part of the Closing-down Procedure keeps your energy field strong and protects you by not allowing the entry of incompatible energies.

EXERCISE 18

The Sphere of Protection

- Still standing relaxed and breathing naturally, knees gently flexed, surround the sphere of coloured light (as in the previous exercise) with a sphere of golden light. See the golden sphere sparkle and gleam. This will tell you about its energy of strength and protection. Spend a moment of awareness before moving from your place.

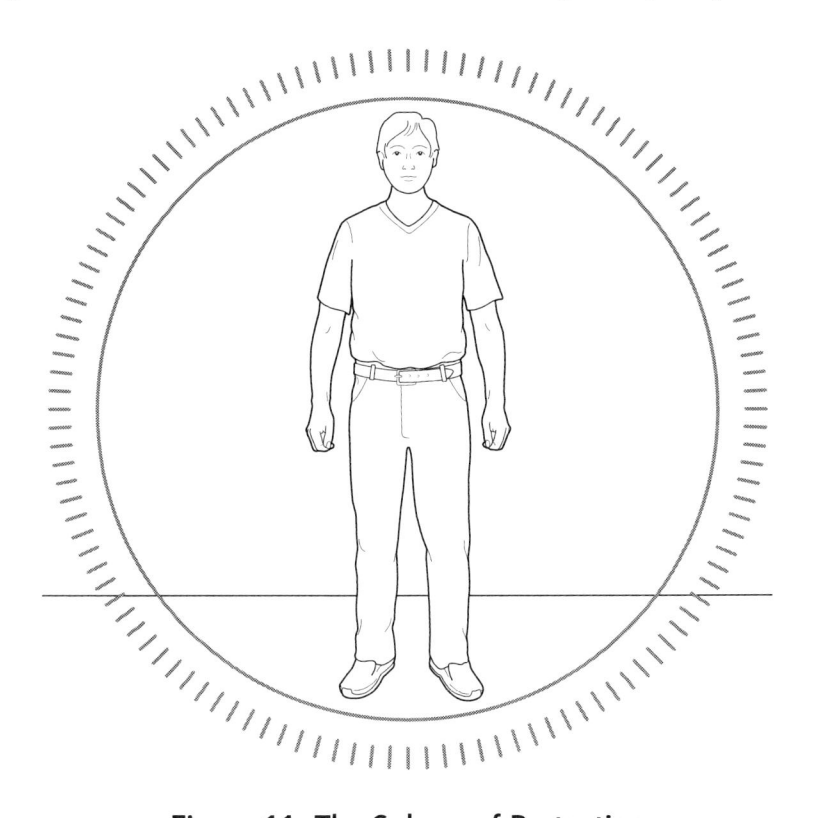

Figure 11. The Sphere of Protection

exercise continues ▶

- The Sphere of Protection can also be used at any time when you wish to protect or maintain the integrity of your energy field, such as when travelling, going shopping, being with crowds, being with individuals or in situations where the energies seem incompatible with your own. You can also use it at the end of the day before sleep.

Your complete baseline practice

The two Distant Healing practices and the Closing-down Procedure are your complete baseline practice. All the other practices of Distant Healing, including the advanced ones, derive from this simple format. This form of focused work brings with it all the benefits of meditation such as reduced blood pressure, a stronger immune system, mental clarity, emotional stability and communication with your Higher Self. These are not reasons for doing Distant Healing, but they are its positive and welcome by-products. Similarly, the Closing-down Procedure reminds you that part of the work is to look after yourself and your energy field.

Chapter 6

Baseline practice – the healing circle

The group experience

However much we might enjoy working solo we are always aware that we are actually working with at least one other person. This person links us to society and the global family. Humans thrive in community. Therefore, if it is possible, I recommend that you join with another or others on a regular basis to do Distant Healing as a group. This not only provides you with the benefits of company and friendship; you will have a forum for learning and feedback, and the experience of building, and being part of, a group energy. This energy is different to that you will experience working alone and it will provide further valuable experience as a Distant Healer.

I hope there will come a time when Distant Healing groups are set up all over the world, in every town and in every country. The energy of a like-minded group is particularly effective in creating favourable conditions for Distant Healing. The Distant Healing Circle provides an opportunity to do service for the community and the wider world, and the basics of the work can be learned almost straight away. The format below is a suggested guideline that can be adapted according to numbers and preferences.

You will need a group leader/facilitator each time you meet and every member should take a turn at this. As in the two baseline exercises for individual work, the group can practise these, as follows. Bring either a list of requests for healing or a list of those who have intuitively come to mind. The length of your list will be dictated by the time you have together. A list of about ten should be enough.

> **EXERCISE 19**
>
> ## *The Distant Healing Circle – sending out the healing Light*
>
> Disconnect all telephones. Have a circle of chairs in the centre of which is a small table with a candle and some matches. Members might like to add items symbolising healing, and so on. Where possible, the group should sit with male next to female, experienced next to inexperienced. By alternating genders, the energies of the circle are easier to balance. This also applies to alternating experienced with inexperienced members.
>
> The chosen leader should open the meeting with a welcome, help the group to attune and then facilitate the Distant Healing. Make sure that everyone has their list of people, animals, situations, etc.
>
> - The group members sit in a circle with feet flat on the floor, and the hands, palms up, on their thighs, or in their laps without linking. The leader instructs the group as follows:
>
> - 'Take six breaths to calm and relax the body, letting go of any worries or anxieties with the out-breath, through the open mouth. Close the mouth, when you feel attuned, and breathe normally.
>
> - 'Check that the body is relaxed, including the back of the neck, the shoulders and pelvis. Close your eyes and allow the calm silence to settle on our Circle.'
>
> - The leader lights the candle and dedicates the light to the work of the Circle, asking for protection and soul guidance.
>
> - The leader continues: 'The light of the candle is the Light of the Source of healing. Breathe it into the heart centre. Allow the Light to fill your chest.
>
> *exercise continues* ▶

- 'Now pass the energy in your heart centre to the person on your left so that you are all linked together.' Intuitively, you may have to wait a moment to gather your heart energy before you can pass on.

- The leader should be aware of this and allow enough time for group linking, for this is the foundation of the Circle. With practice, it is possible to sense when energetic linking is complete.

- The leader expresses the purpose of the meeting and gives thanks, on behalf of the group, for the opportunity to be of service.

- The leader begins to read out his or her list, asking for healing Light to be sent to each person named. A simple form of this could be: 'I ask for healing to be sent to (name).' The leader indicates that the list is complete with a verbal signal such as 'Thank you.'

- The person on the leader's left then reads out the next list and repeats the concluding signal. Follow this procedure until everyone has read out their list.

- With your eyes closed, you can create an inner 'screen' (just above the brow) on which you may be able to 'see' the people named. It is important to know that your intention, motivated by love, has enabled the light of healing to be sent to them.

- As you sit together in the silence, the leader gives time for quiet reflection.

- After a short break, the group can discuss the work of the Circle, share experiences and queries to consolidate learning.

- The work may be followed by another spiritual activity such as meditation, a reading, or listening to music.

- Finally, the leader closes the Healing Circle. As the candle is blown out, the Light can be sent out to where it is needed, as when working alone – to a strife-ridden place, an environment under threat, and so on.

exercise continues ▶

- Before closing the meeting, the group should carry out the Closing-down Procedure. This could be led by the chosen leader.

The reflection time can be used to make notes, or illustrate the experience in some way. This allows the group members to log their experience and learning, chart the energies they have been working with and ground the experience. It gives the mind time to absorb what has happened, which is one of the building blocks of group work.

Members can devise activities for coming together as a group. These should help members to leave behind the life they lead outside the meeting place. I have suggested a format above, but there can be different types of group activity. For example, the group leader for a particular meeting could suggest the topic for group activity, such as a local, national or global crisis. This utilises the group's ability to channel energy to such situations, rather than to the individual list.

The group can alternate sending out the Light with the second baseline technique for group work: creating the Light column.

EXERCISE 20
The Distant Healing Circle – creating the Light column

Disconnect all telephones. Have a circle of chairs in the centre of which is a small table with a candle and some matches. Members might like to add items symbolising healing, and so on. Where possible, the group should sit with male next to female, experienced next to inexperienced. By alternating genders, the energies of the Circle are easier to balance. This also applies to alternating experienced with inexperienced members.

The chosen leader should open the meeting with a welcome, help the group to attune, and then facilitate the Distant Healing. Make sure that everyone has their list of people, animals, situations, etc.

exercise continues ▶

- The group members sit in a circle with feet flat on the floor, and the hands, palms up, on their thighs, or in their laps without linking. The leader instructs the group as follows:

- 'Take six breaths to calm and relax the body, letting go of any worries or anxieties (which may be uppermost in your mind since compiling your list) with the out-breath, through the open mouth. Close your mouth, when you feel attuned, and breathe normally.

- 'Check that the body is relaxed, including the back of the neck, the shoulders and pelvis. Close your eyes and allow the calm silence to settle on our Circle.'

- The leader lights the candle and dedicates the Light to the work of the Circle, asking for protection and soul guidance.

- 'The light of the candle is the Light of the Source of healing. Breathe it into the heart centre. Allow the Light to fill your chest.'

- 'Now pass the energy in your heart centre to the person on your left so that you are all linked together.' Intuitively, you may have to wait a moment to gather your heart energy before you can pass on.

- The leader should be aware of this and allow enough time for group linking, for this is the foundation of the circle. With practice, it is possible to sense when energetic linking is complete.

- The leader expresses the purpose of the meeting and gives thanks, on behalf of the group, for the opportunity to be of service. The leader continues:

- 'As you are aware of the Light in the heart centre, in your mind's eye see this light extending from you to the centre of the Circle.' In this way every member helps to build a central column of Light, the Light of healing.

exercise continues ▶

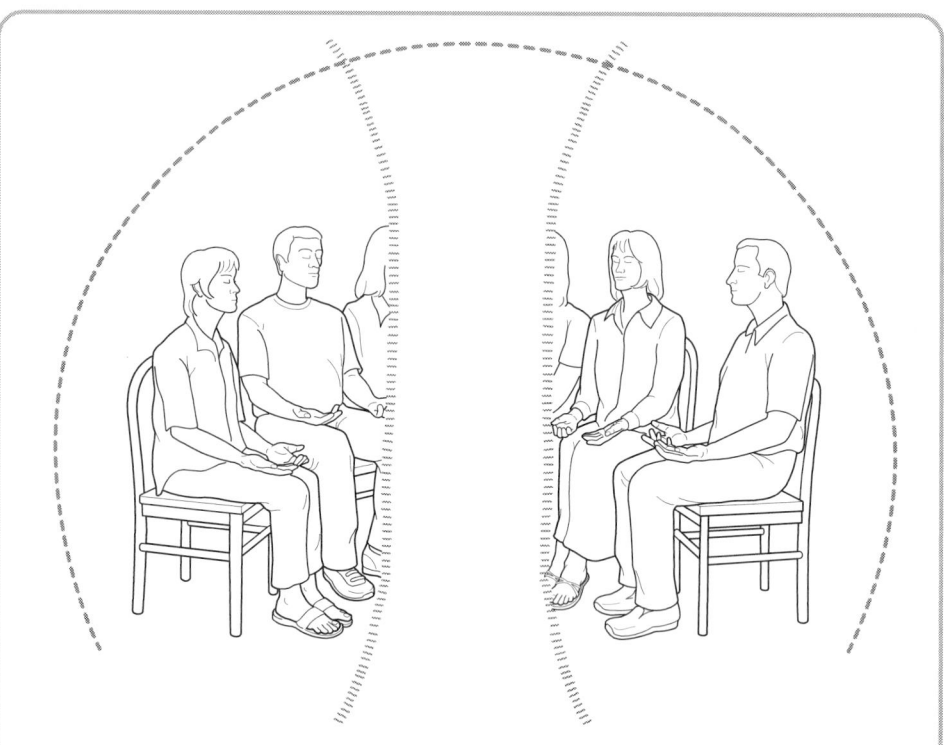

Figure 12. The Distant Healing Circle – creating the Light column

- The leader begins to read out the first list, asking for healing for each person named, knowing that they will be put or held in the Light. A simple form of this could be: 'I ask for healing for (name).' The leader indicates that the list is complete with a verbal signal such as 'Thank you.'

- The person on the leader's left then reads out the next list and repeats the concluding signal. Follow this procedure until everyone has read out their list.

- By watching your inner 'screen' (above the brow), you may be able to 'see' the people named, or you may not. It is important to know that your intention, motivated by love, has put them in the Light of healing.

- As you sit together in the silence, retain your awareness of the Light. See if your inner screen shows you what is happening to the Light.

exercise continues ▶

- The leader gives time for quiet reflection.

- After a short break, the group can discuss the work of the Circle, share experiences and queries to consolidate learning.

- The work may be followed by another spiritual activity such as meditation, a reading, or listening to music.

- Finally, the leader closes the Healing Circle. As the candle is blown out, the light can be sent out to where it is needed, as when working alone.

- Before closing the meeting, the group should carry out the Closing-down Procedure. This could be led by the chosen leader.

As before, the reflection time can be used to make notes, or illustrate the experience in some way. This allows the group members to log their experience and learning, chart the energies they have been working with, and ground the experience. It gives the mind time to absorb what has happened, which is one of the building blocks of group work.

Members can devise activities for coming together as a group. These should help them to leave behind the life they lead outside the meeting place. I have suggested a format above, but there can be different types of group activity. For example, the group leader for a particular meeting could suggest the topic for group activity, such as a local, national or global crisis. This utilises the group's ability to channel energy to such situations, rather than to the individual list.

Moving on to Part Two

When you, and your Distant Healing Circle, feel confident with your practice so far, you are ready to move forward with the topics in Part Two.

Beginning with important information about the body's subtle energy circuits and the energy centres, Part Two also looks at how we are affected both by our Distant Healing work and the effects of negative energies in general. This is followed by the advanced techniques for solo and group work. As well as strengthening your traditional practice with persons and animals, your work with Part Two will also equip you to make a valuable contribution to global healing.

＃ *Part Two*

Chapter 7

The energy circuits of the body

The polarity channels of the etheric body

On each side of the central channel, and connected to it, are two further channels which extend from the base to the brow centres.

The circulation of energy in the two channels creates a balance between the inflow and outflow of subtle energies throughout the system, including each of the centres.

The polarities of energy have been historically referred to as 'masculine' and 'feminine', based on the relative roles of male and female in procreation, but they describe qualities of energy flow not aspects of gender. Everyone has both channels and both energies. The emissive, right side of the field processes energies that are outgoing. The receptive, left side processes energies that are incoming.

For emotional and mental health, as well as physical well-being, the energies of the two polarities should be in a state of balance, but it is easy for them to get out of balance. Our mental or emotional state, our thoughts or behaviour, have an instant effect on this balance. For example, when we are not assertive enough in a given situation, so that we allow ourselves to be disempowered, the emissive energies are not being used when they need to be. The polarities are either thrown out of balance or their imbalance has caused us to be unable to stand up for ourselves. We then experience feelings such as anger, frustration or self-disgust, which are warning us about the energetic outcome. If this goes on for too long so that one energy stream is unused or underdeveloped, the other will try to

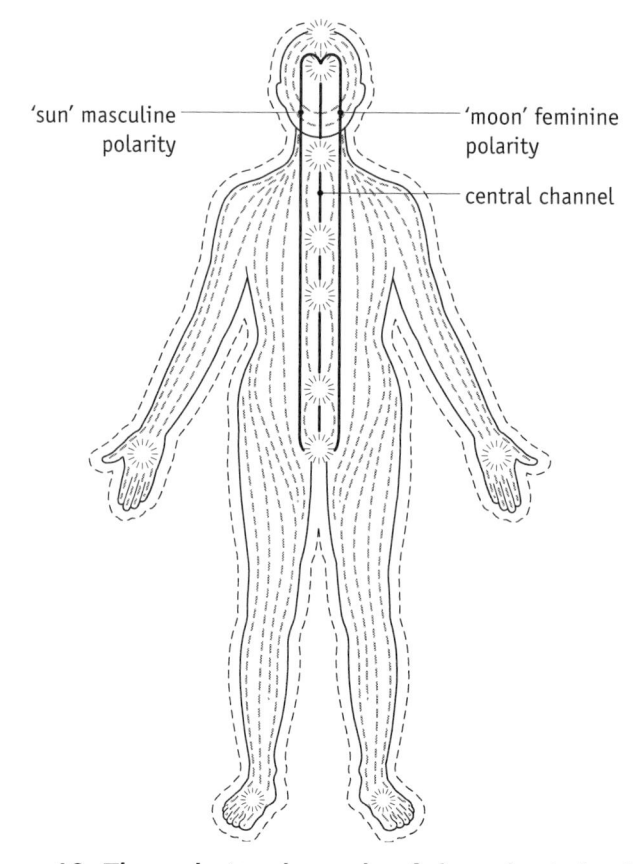

Figure 13. The polarity channels of the etheric body

compensate by dominating the system and all its activities. This is self-defeating since it nurtures the initial weakness.

Experience will tell you when your healing work is involved in restoring polarity balance (see also Exercise 23: Checking polarity balance, page 78).

The template for the body

The template for the formation, development and composition of the physical body is found in the etheric body. Thus, the symmetry of the body is derived from the symmetry of the etheric, with its central channel and network of energy centres. The body's ability to process the flow of substances to and from its organs is derived from the flow of energies in the etheric channels. The seven main energy centres are the structures from which the seven endocrine glands are derived. Other physical organs originate in other large energy centres. The nervous system is derived from the system of etheric energy channels and the vascular (blood) system from the flow of energies within the etheric network. The fact that we can absorb subtle energies through the skin is due to the presence of tiny energy centres throughout the surface of the etheric body. These foundations of the physical body have a direct bearing on how and whether healing energies flow into it from a spiritual level.

Throughout the existence of the body, the etheric conveys the life force, essential to the animation of all physical forms, along with vitalising energies which enter via the sacral and solar plexus centres. In this way, the etheric is the energetic support system for physical life. This gateway between the physical and the non-physical is the entry level for the Higher Self and its subtle energies into physical life.

We are beings of Light

It is essential to realise that we are first and foremost conscious beings of Light, manifestations of the Oneness. The Light being, or soul, originates its own subtle aspects (mental, emotional and etheric) which support and make possible the life of the physical. We are then able to develop an individual personality consciousness from the time of conception onwards.

As we have all experienced, the problem with our personality consciousness is that it can easily convince us that *it* is the real 'us'. It is only the pressure from our Higher Self, or soul, that encourages us to consider that we have a far greater consciousness. All this does mean, however, that when the personality becomes unconscious, as it does during sleep and at death, the Higher Self withdraws from the physical and we move into consciousness at some subtle level.

The skeleton and its subtle energies

For the body to act as the soul's travelling vehicle it needs a structure that will provide a strong, rigid, yet movable base. This is the physical role of the skeleton. This symmetrical structure has a central flexible column, the spine, which protects the central nervous system. The spine is topped by the skull, which houses and protects the brain – the 'computer' of all the body systems. The spine supports the two girdles of the shoulders and pelvis, from which hang the bones of the arms and legs. The rib cage, emanating from the spine and joined in front by the breast bone, houses and protects the heart, lungs, stomach, liver and associated organs.

Etheric consciousness is aware of the energetic state of the bones through the subtle energy circuits of the skeleton. In the illustration below these are indicated in black for clarity but they should be visualised as fine lines of light.

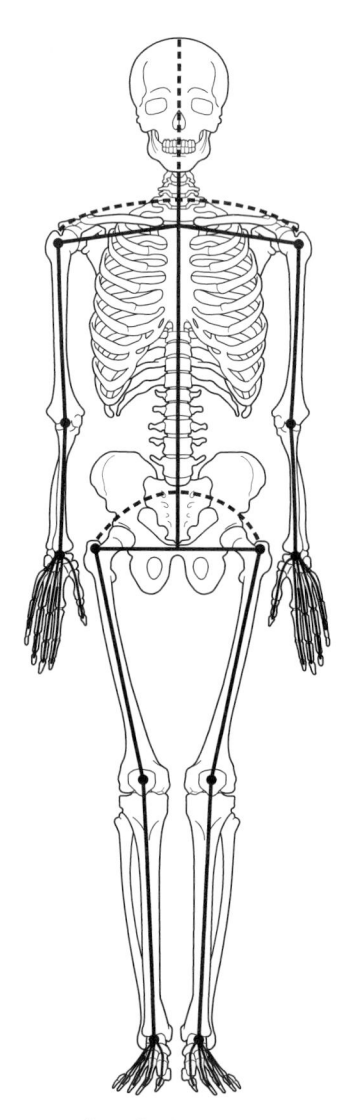

Figure 14. The skeletal energy circuits

The bones carry information about where a person is on their life journey. They are also our link with the mineral kingdom and its Earth memory.

Since your work may well involve the skeletal energy circuits, the following exercises will introduce you to them. You will need a partner and, if possible, a healing couch or a means of working with your partner lying down. There is also an exercise with your partner sitting on a chair.

EXERCISE 21
Sensing the skeletal energy circuits

Having looked again at the diagram of the skeleton, your intention is to make contact with the skeletal energy circuits, with your palm centres acting as scanning sensors. This is done by holding your hands, palms down, 5–10cm (2–4in) above your partner's body. The subtle energies of the skeleton radiate beyond the physical body. Thus it is perfectly possible to scan the spine from above. In hands-on healing, this fact enables the healer to work with patients who are unable to lie on the front of their body.

You will first scan down the primary circuit of the spine, then down the secondary circuits of one side – the shoulder girdle and the arm, the pelvis and the leg. Then scan down the secondary circuits of the other side, with the spine as the starting point of each secondary circuit. Your partner should lie on his or her back, relaxing and breathing normally. At all times follow the form of the skeleton. You may find it helpful to have a practice run to get used to the procedure. Note your sensations at each part of the scanning and sensing.

- Stand by your partner's head and hold both palms about 5–10cm (2–4in) away from the top of the skull. Keep a small gap between your two hands. Move them slowly over the skull and down over the face towards the neck, to sense where the spine links with the

exercise continues ▶

skull. This is where your primary scan of the spine begins. With your hands 5–10cm (2–4in) above the front of the body, move your hands slowly from the neck, following the line of the spine, until you reach its base at the coccyx. Leave one hand here while you extend the other back to the top of the spine. As you stand with your arms extended, see if you can sense the energy of the spine between your two palms.

- To move down the left side of your partner's body, put both palms opposite the base of the neck, keeping a slight gap between them, as before. Move them slowly to the top of the left shoulder. Continue slowly down the arm, from joint to joint, until you are able to move out over the hand and the bones of the fingers. Leave one hand here while you extend the other to the top of the left shoulder. Again, see if you can sense the energy of the left arm between your palms.

- Now scan the left leg. Put your hands opposite the base of the spine. Move them slowly across the pelvis to the left hip. Continue slowly down the left leg, from joint to joint, until you are able to move out over the bones of the toes. Leave one hand there while you extend the other back to the hip. See if you can sense the energy of the left leg.

- Scan down the right side of your partner's skeleton in the same way, beginning where the shoulder girdle meets the spine.

- When you have completed your scan of the energy circuits of the skeleton, discuss your impressions with your partner. Change roles. Finally, compare notes with each other.

If you would prefer to work with your partner sitting on a chair, try the next exercise. Read through the one above so that you are acquainted with its method and purpose.

EXERCISE 22
Sensing the skeletal energy circuits – partner on a chair

- Your partner should sit with feet flat on the ground with the legs uncrossed and hands resting on the thighs. The palms may be up or down. Relax and breathe normally. Stand behind your partner with your own palms held 5–10cm (2–4in) away from the back of the skull, with a slight gap between them. Move them slowly down the back of the skull towards the neck until you sense where the skull joins the spine. This is where your primary scan of the spine begins.

- Move your palms slowly down the spine until they are opposite its base at the coccyx. Leave one hand here while you extend the other to the top of the spine. As in the previous exercise, see if you can feel the energy of the spine between your two palms.

- To move down the left side of your partner's body, put both palms at the back of the neck. Move them slowly across to the top of the left shoulder. Continue down the left arm, joint by joint, until you are able to move out over the bones of the fingers. Leave one hand here while you extend the other to the top of the arm. Sense the energy of the left arm.

- Now scan the left leg. Standing behind the back, put your palms opposite the base of the spine. Move them slowly across the pelvis to the left. Continue down the left leg, joint by joint, until you are able to move out over the bones of the left foot. Leave one hand here while you extend the other to the top of the leg. Sense the energy of the left leg.

- Scan the right side in the same way. Begin with both palms at the base of the neck to scan the right arm. Return to the base of the spine to scan the right leg.

exercise continues ▶

- When you have completed your scan of the skeletal energy circuits, discuss your findings with your partner. Change roles. Finally, compare notes with each other.

The symmetry of the skeleton and its energy circuits reflect the polarity energy channels in the etheric, as shown earlier (Figures 13 and 14, pages 72 and 74). They facilitate the balance of energy flow in the skeleton, muscles and their skeletal attachments. This means that the system seeks to ensure the proper movement of the limbs and their joints, and the efficient mobility of the whole structure.

From a Distant Healing point of view, the energy circuits also offer a way in to those energies that are needed to bring balance to a person's being at every level. You may find, therefore, that in some aspect of your work, you are working to restore polarity balance. The next exercise will make you familiar with this procedure.

EXERCISE 23
Checking polarity balance

In this exercise you will use the soles of the feet as well as the tops of the shoulders to sense the energetic polarity balance of the skeleton.

- Your partner should lie on the healing couch or on the ground. Position yourself by your partner's feet with your palms 5–10cm (2–4in) away from the soles. Relax and breathe normally. See if you can sense the energies emanating from them. Do both feet feel the same?

- Do you sense energy *leaving* your palms? If so, this is to restore energetic balance. When this is the case, both feet will feel the same energetically.

- What was your partner aware of?

exercise continues ▶

- Change roles and compare notes. Try this second part of the exercise on another day.
- Position yourself at your partner's head. Hold your palms near the tops of your partner's shoulders and repeat the above procedures. What did you sense and what was your partner aware of?
- Again, compare your findings.

EXERCISE 24

Checking polarity balance – partner on a chair

- This is the same exercise as above. Your partner should sit on the chair, legs uncrossed, with the feet flat on the ground. The hands should rest on the thighs. Relax and breathe normally. Squat by your partner's feet and hold your palms near the tops of them. See if you can sense the energies emanating from them. Do both feet feel the same?
- Do you sense energy *leaving* your palms, to bring balance, so that both feet eventually feel the same energetically?
- What was your partner aware of?
- Change roles and compare notes. Try this second part of the exercise on another day.
- Stand behind your partner and hold your palms near the tops of your partner's shoulders and repeat the above procedures. What did you sense and what was your partner aware of?
- Compare your findings.

You are building a concept of a human being that will form a base for your Distant Healing work. You are beginning to discover that there is much more to you than your physical body. By realising that your body is the expression of your soul's need to experience physical life, you celebrate your discoveries.

Distant Healing acknowledges the essential *spiritual* nature of all energy. The reality of our body of Light is made possible through its subtle energies. In the next chapter we look at the etheric structures that facilitate energetic flow, and every aspect of our life and journey. These are the etheric gateways: the subtle energy centres (chakras).

Chapter 8

Etheric gateways – the subtle energy centres

THERE ARE SOME 360 centres discernible in the etheric body, varying in size and function. Distant Healing is particularly concerned with the seven main energy centres because they act as the gateways, and gatekeepers, of our life journey, our health and well-being.

For these reasons, do not attempt to shut off their activity by 'closing' them. While specific processes are going on in each centre, the system operates as a complete and interconnected whole and, through etheric consciousness, each centre is aware of all the activities in the system.

The main centres appear as slight depressions in the luminous weblike surface of the etheric body. Each is attached to a central channel, aligned with the spine, which is in turn connected to the network of channels running through the etheric (Figure 7, page 33). During the operation of a centre, the vortex of light moves out from the surface of the etheric body to project into the energy field. It now appears as a bell- or funnel-shaped structure connected at its narrower end to the central channel. This shape facilitates the gathering or emission of energies.

The etheric effectively acts as the communication vehicle for the soul, enabling the passage of energies from the Higher Self (soul) to the physical and from the physical back to the Higher Self. In doing so, the centres act as a distribution system for all the energies, including the mental and emotional, generated during life experience. Throughout these activities, the centres identify subtle energies and, if possible, process them. But very often a person is not ready to deal with a certain situation, such as

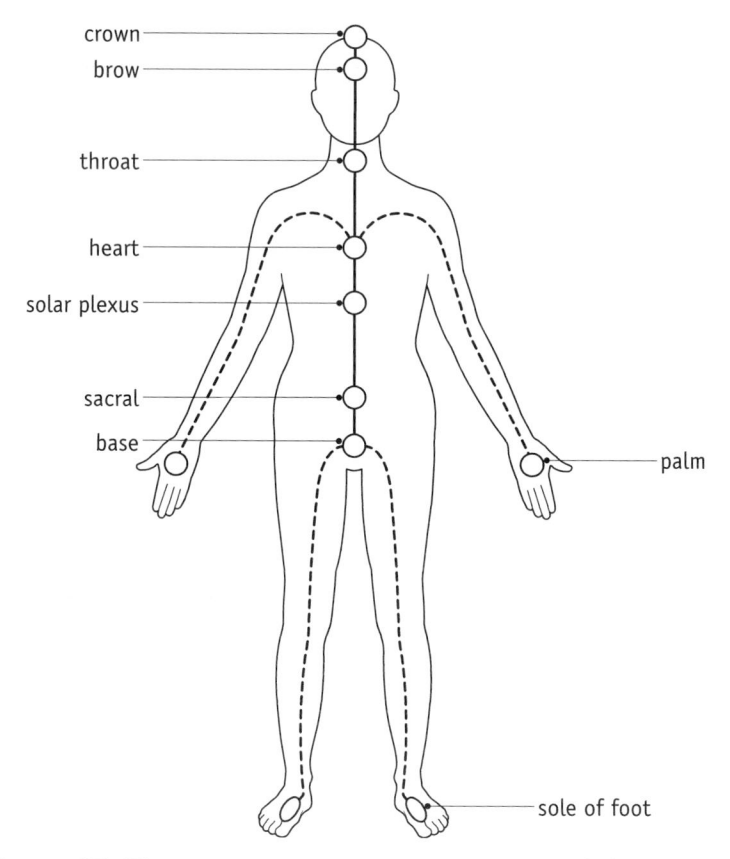

Figure 15. The seven main energy centres and the centres of the hands and feet

bereavement, and the etheric consciousness stores the relevant energies for processing later.

However, if unprocessed material is allowed to build up, we begin to receive warning signals from the Higher Self, in the form of uncomfortable feelings. If these are not heeded, the body may become sick so that we are forced to 'listen'.

Similarly, whenever a person confronts a situation contrary to the personal spiritual core, the centres work hard to process the material. But continued exposure makes this progressively more difficult, which can exhaust the centres and lead to energetic blockage and subsequent ill-health.

EXERCISE 25
Sensing the location of the centres

You will need a partner for this exercise. Have another look at Figure 15, page 82, so that you have a fair idea where you will be working in this exercise. Take your time and pause between locating each centre if you need to.

- Your partner should be seated on a chair with legs and arms uncrossed (if they remain crossed there is an energy block at the point of crossover), feet flat on the ground, hands resting on the thighs. Your partner should relax and breathe normally.

- Remember to use your breath to help you to stay relaxed as your mind starts to collate the subtle energy information that you are tracing.

- Stand behind your partner and raise your hands up so that your palms can be held above your partner's crown centre with your arms fully extended. Keep a small gap between your hands.

- Slowly lower your arms, allowing your palms to move down towards your partner's crown centre until you sense a slight pressure or resistance against your palms. Stop at this point. Notice your own sensations.

- This is the edge of the radiation you can sense from the crown centre. Notice where the crown centre energies extend upwards into the energy field.

- Now you are going to sense the location of the brow centre. Here, the energies project in front of and behind the centre so you will need to step to one side of your partner while you move your hands to either side of the brow centre with your arms extended.

exercise continues ▶

84 • THE DISTANT HEALING HANDBOOK

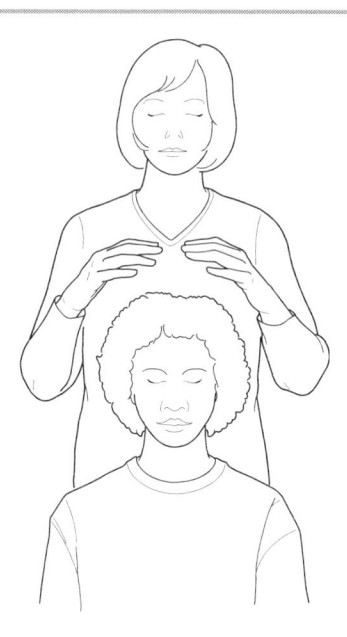

Figure 16. Sensing the crown centre

- Slowly bring both your palms in towards the brow centre until you feel the slight pressure of its projected energies. Stop at this point and notice where the brow energies extend into the field. Notice any sensations and any differences in sensations.

- Move both hands down to the throat area. Again, extend your arms away from the throat and slowly bring them together to locate the energies of the throat centre.

- Move both hands down to the centre of your partner's chest. Again, with one hand in front and the other behind with your arms extended. Slowly bring them together to locate the heart centre.

- Move both hands down to just below your partner's breast bone, above the navel. Keep both arms extended. Slowly bring them together to locate the solar plexus centre. You may find that you need to kneel on the ground or use another chair to sit on so that you are comfortable while working with the lower centres. It is important to relax to be fully sensitive.

exercise continues ▶

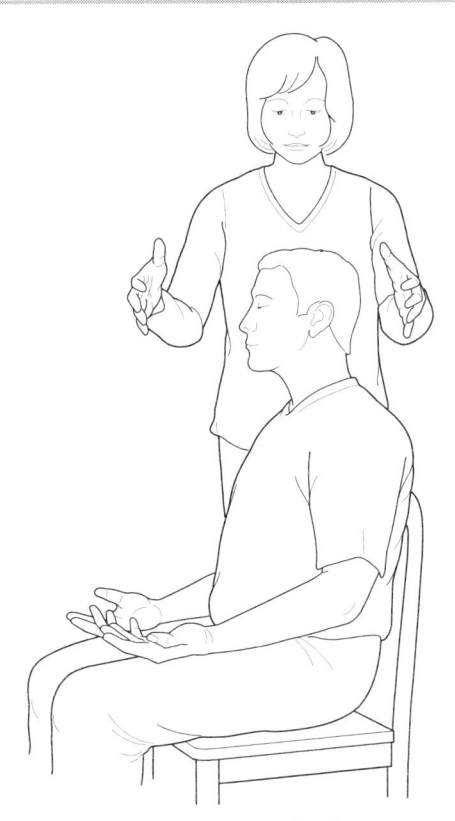

Figure 17. Sensing the brow centre

- Move both hands just below your partner's navel to locate the sacral centre. Keep both arms extended. Slowly bring them together. Again, check your sensations and mentally compare them with those of the other centres.

- Finally, to the base centre. When a person is in a sitting position, the base centre energies project upwards and downwards at an angle of about 45 degrees. Position yourself so that your palms are held at this angle.

- Proceed in the same way as for the other centres to sense the energies of the base centre.

- Relax and, after a short break, change roles. Finally, compare notes with your partner.

Figure 18. Sensing the base centre

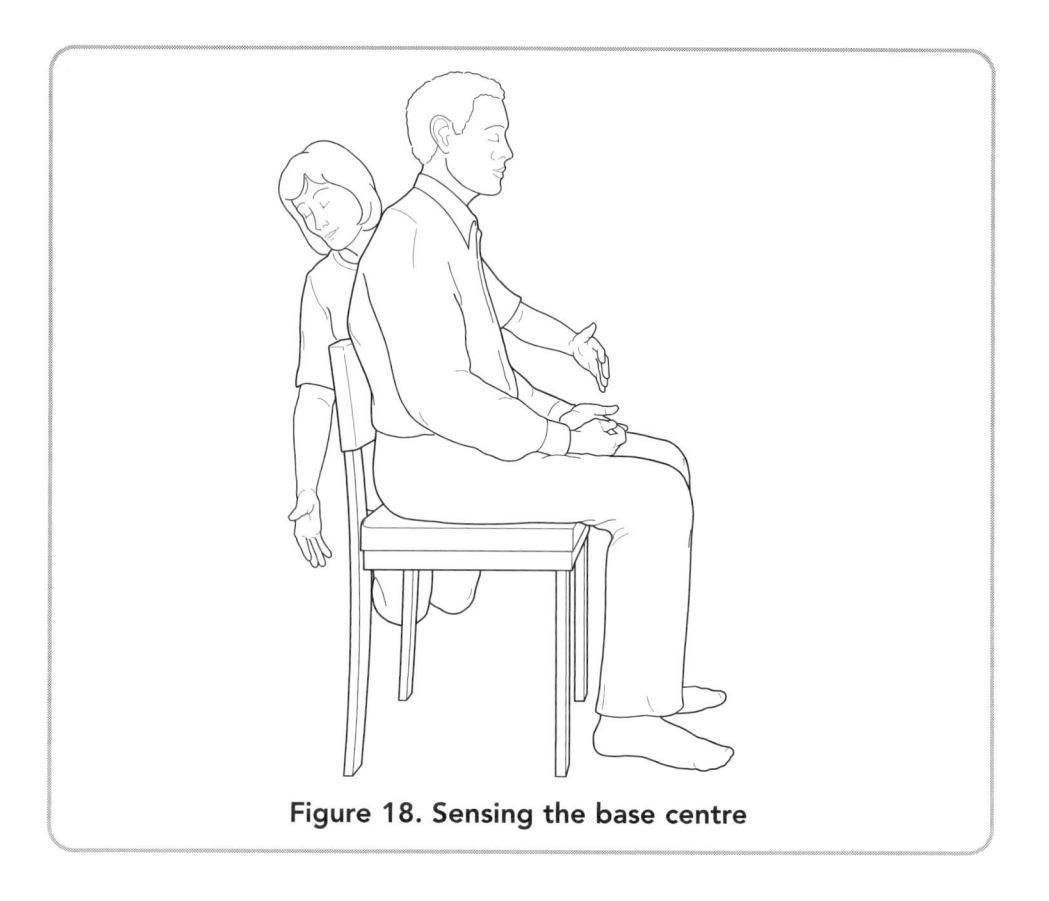

That exercise helped you to locate the energies of the centres and showed you how your palm centres were sensitive to them. Now we can look at the life issues that each of them is processing. The material presented here is based on my own research over some 25 years and has been found to apply to all my patients and to all workshop participants. It is offered as a starting point for your own experience and awareness.

The seven major centres are located near major organs in the body, some of which are nerve plexuses. As we shall see, each of the major centres deals energetically with specific life issues – survival, sexuality, love, for example. The energies of these processes move in and out of the body via seven endocrine glands (the glands without ducts). In this way, life issues can have an impact on our body, starting at a glandular level and then moving into nearby organs.

Similarly, what happens to our body is conveyed energetically to the relevant centre or centres. To give a simple example: a person experiences the loss of a loved one and soon develops a severe cold. This is because the immune system, via the thymus gland, is linked to the heart centre, which deals with all issues concerning love. The feelings of grief have manifested as a shock to the immune system, leaving the person vulnerable to infection.

Below is an outline of the work of the seven life gateways. We will move in the same direction as the evolutionary force of the centre energies: from the base to the crown. Remember, the centres are *etheric* structures. They operate through the relevant endocrine glands, wherever these happen to be physically situated.

The base centre

Located at the base of the spine, this centre is our link with our body, nature, the planet and the element earth. It processes all issues of a physical nature: how we relate to our body and its physicality; the senses; sensuality; the sex or gender that we are (and remember there are two polarities of male and female, with many variations on those themes); our safety and survival; self-defence and aggression; how we relate to all aspects of the natural world; how we relate to the planet. As you can see, these basic issues are all related to being here and, energetically, have to be accepted and dealt with.

The base centre links with the body via the adrenal glands on the top of the kidneys. These are the glands that get things moving, and they are also concerned with our self-defence: to 'fight or flight'. Interestingly, people who have issues around personal safety, especially children, often have skin problems which affect their hands. If you look at a person with the hands held by the sides of the body, the hands are seen to be aligned with the base centre. Thus, base centre issues, such as survival, can erupt on the hands as a warning sign that things are not as they should be.

This centre is also concerned with the base of the spine, the lower pelvis and related organs, the hips, legs and feet. It is the keeper of cellular memory for the whole body.

When in a state of balance, the centre vibrates to the colour red. Like all centre colours, it is seen with subtle vision and is similar to, but not identical with, the colours of the physical spectrum. Balance occurs when a person feels safe and secure, and has a good relationship with the body and the natural world.

The base centre has a special link with the heart and crown centres. This link gives a strong clue about our reality. The base centre emphasises that we are in a physical body in a physical world, but our nature is love (heart centre) and our origins are spiritual (crown centre).

The sacral centre

Located opposite the sacral bones in the spine, between the navel and the base centre, this centre processes all issues of creativity and sexuality (how we express ourselves sexually). It links us with the element of water. The 'inner child' is originally located here. It keeps a subtle energetic record of our development as a child. When a person has experienced childhood trauma, however, the inner child is often found misplaced in either the base or solar plexus centres.

The sacral is the seat of joy, which is not simply an emotion but an energy generated by this centre, telling us that we are in touch with its spiritual aspects. Not surprisingly, this is often expressed in the form of giggly laughter, especially in children. Being human is to have the potential to be creative in some way (this is a natural manifestation of our unique divinity). Thus suppression of creativity, or sexuality, creates issues that have to be processed by this centre. A useful question when we need to assess how we really feel about something is: Does it give me joy?

The sacral centre is linked to the body via the sex glands (usually the testes in the male or the ovaries in the female). It is concerned with the urogenital organs, the uterus (womb), the kidneys, the lower digestive organs and the lower back. Males should realise that they may not have a physical uterus, but they do have a sacral centre that acts like one. All creations have their beginnings and gestation here.

When in a state of balance, the sacral vibrates to the colour orange. But when our creativity is not expressed the centre moves out of balance and begins to find ways to signal this.

The sacral centre has a special link with the throat centre, where creativity is given expression.

The solar plexus centre

Just below the breast bone and the diaphragm, above the navel, the nerve junction known as the solar plexus gives this centre its name. The nerves of this plexus radiate out like the rays of the sun and echo its subtle activity pattern in the etheric centre. This is where we sense nervous feelings like 'butterflies in the stomach' that can impact on the diaphragm to affect our breathing. It has these physical effects because it is linked to the body via the islets of Langerhans: the endocrine glands in the pancreas. Its energies affect the digestive system, the pancreas, the liver and gall bladder, the diaphragm and middle back.

The processing of our thoughts, emotions and feelings, our sense of personal self and personal power is generated by this centre. Here we discover how far life experience has empowered or disempowered us, and how we react to people and situations in terms of our sense of self. As we have grown, developed, experienced life and reacted to the behaviour of others, this sense of self has been created by our mind. We should understand, then, that our personality, which embodies our sense of self, is a conditioned being. The unconditioned being that watches over us without any kind of judgement, and is present at all times, is our Higher Self.

The solar plexus centre confronts us with all issues connected to the mind, our thoughts and emotions, especially our conditioned mindsets. The mind is designed to record and remember, and this process begins in, and continues from, our time in the womb. Since some of our experience will inevitably be 'negative', we find that not all of our mind's conditioning is conducive to our well-being.

The solar plexus centre allows us to store mental and emotional patterns of energy which, because they have not been fully processed, can trigger reactions we would rather not experience. This is when we are in danger of moving into a state of energetic imbalance and our feelings tell us how uncomfortable this is.

This is important when considering the link with the brow centre. Though the solar plexus centre processes mental activity, it has access to the intuitive, or soul, information that comes from the brow. Thus we are able to compare and contrast these two related forms of information. But so often we listen to the overriding voice of the mind. For example, have you ever had an idea about something; it seems a good idea and then you start to think it over? You end up changing your mind, only to find later that your first impulse was the best one.

We become conditioned by the rationality of the mind to trust its findings above all else. What we need to remember is that the mind can only work with what it already knows: with what is in the memory bank. Material from the brow is always fresh and often 'unknown' so that when the mind is confronted with such material it tends to advise against using it.

In its balanced state, the solar plexus centre vibrates to the colour golden yellow.

These first three centres of the system are very much concerned with being physically human and having a human life. The energies moving upwards from them next enter the heart centre, where they will be assessed to see how much they have been associated with unconditional love.

The heart centre

Located in the centre of the chest *not* the physical heart, this is considered the place of the soul. The challenge of the heart centre is to express the light of the soul as love, to get its soul message of love through to us and to deal with all issues about love, and lovelessness, in our life.

The heart centre links to the body via the thymus gland. This endocrine gland is quite large when we are very young and tends to diminish in size as we get older. It is linked with the development of the immune system. At a subtle level this continues to be its work, in spite of its physically diminished size, so that issues of love and lovelessness affect our immune system throughout life. This is one of the ways that the heart centre signals to us.

The cardiac and pulmonary nerve plexuses, the heart, lungs, the bronchial tubes, chest, upper back and arms are all influenced by the heart centre. Similarly, information about what happens to these organs passes to other levels of our being via this centre.

I mentioned earlier how the energies of the centres can affect the surrounding, or nearby, organs. An interesting and unusual example of this can occur with the hands because of the energetic link between the heart and base centres. When the arms are held at the sides of the body, the hands are in line with the base centre. The hands can manifest conditions triggered by love and/or lovelessness (heart centre) and survival (base centre). Such conditions include eczema and arthritis.

As can be seen from the illustration (Figure 15, page 82), the heart is at the balance point of the seven main centres so that this is one of its important functions. It has to balance the 'physical' energies moving upwards towards the brow with the 'spiritual' energies moving downwards from the crown. In all cases the heart centre is monitoring how much the conditioned personality is involved, how much the Higher Self is involved, and the balance between them. When in a state of balance it vibrates to the colour green. This is the colour of balance. It is not surprising that when we need to revive and refresh ourselves we go somewhere in nature, unconsciously seeking the energies of the colour green.

We are living in a time when this balance point of the centres is also the crisis point in human affairs. If you think back, you will find that some issue around love has been your greatest life challenge so far. It will continue to be so for all people on the planet. Via the heart centre, the Higher Self asks: Do you love yourself and do you love others as the Source? Do you love others because of Oneness and can you love without judging them? Your heart knows and cannot be fooled.

But these questions are also about whether we are at last willing to move from a fear-based to a love-based way of being. The fear-based way keeps us in the solar plexus centre, in the grip of the conditioned mind. We know what fear would do – fear trusts power and violence. We have had thousands of years of trying this way to solve all our problems and we go on with this way in spite of the evidence that it never provides a long-term solution.

This is why the challenge of our times is to move our consciousness to the heart centre. Then we can ask: What would *Love* do? Love will give an answer to any problem, on any occasion. For when the heart is asked the soul replies and shows us the way through. We are guided by the Higher Self and its links with the sacred. Love's answer makes everybody happy and everybody wins.

Distant Healing is a positive response to this challenge from the heart. Where we might have felt helpless in the face of a great need outside ourselves, Distant Healing offers simple ways to bring balance and healing. Love is always dynamic. This is what gives power to the heart energy of compassion, ensuring that our caring response is more than useless pity. Distant Healing can be your way to move to a love-based way of being.

From the point of balance in the subtle energy system, the next centre deals with all aspects of expression and communication. This ranges from expressing who we think we are (our limited and conditioned self-image), and expressing who we really are (our talents and soul mission), to what else is going on in the whole system. It is profoundly influenced by its nearness to the brow centre where intuitive or soul knowledge is generated.

The throat centre

Though located in the throat and affecting its related organs, the throat centre is the 'ear, nose and throat' centre too. It links with the body, and these organs, via the thyroid gland. As mentioned earlier, the throat has an important energetic link with the sacral where everything creative is conceived and gestated.

There is an old wooden grave marker in a cemetery in Arizona on which the epitaph counsels: 'Be what you iz, coz if you be what you aint, then you aint what you iz.' Each centre seems to throw out a challenge to us and that epitaph exactly sums up the challenge of the throat centre: to be authentic. Here are processed all issues of expression and communication, and all the different ways we use to express ourselves and communicate with others, with the world, and the realms of the sacred.

The throat centre asks: Do you express who you really are, or only part of yourself, none of yourself, or a distorted aspect of yourself? Do you value truth or is the lie OK? Untruth accumulates energies like itself, and attracts energies from outside us that are like itself. Gradually whole areas of our being and our life become weighed down with the heavy energies of falsehood and negativity. They have no power to do any good, even though this may have been our motive for lying.

In the other centres it may take time before we are aware of a block in the flow of energies in the system, but if we suppress the *expression* of any of the subtle energies, we feel a pain in the throat, or the need to cough, straight away. I remember as a child being wrongly accused of a misdemeanour and not being allowed to speak up for myself. This created an intense dull pain in the larynx. In this example, not only was expression being denied but also the truth about the situation. Hence, the throat centre is concerned with issues around justice/fairness and injustice/unfairness.

When in a state of balance, the throat centre vibrates to the colour sky blue. This is very often the colour of healing energies as perceived by subtle sensing. If you find yourself suffering from a throat discomfort, like those described above, this can be relieved by visualising that you can breathe a sky-blue-coloured light into the throat. Do this slowly and gently with six breaths, letting go of the pain, and thoughts and feelings about the issue, with the out-breath.

The brow centre

Located in the middle of the forehead, just above the brow, the brow centre links with the body via the pituitary gland and hypothalamus of the brain. It is concerned with the brain, eyes and face. One of the roles of the brow centre is to oversee the operation of the centres below it. When subtle energies arrive here for transmission to the crown, the brow will send them back down the system if they have not been processed (if we have not dealt with the relevant issues).

I described earlier how the physical body is based on the etheric template. A good illustration of this is the way the pituitary gland and hypothalamus mirror the activity of the brow centre by controlling and monitoring the secretions of all the other endocrine glands.

The brow centre processes information from our psychic awareness, or subtle sensing, our so-called 'sixth sense', as well as information from our intuitive awareness, or soul sensing. Both forms of energetic information are passed to the solar plexus centre, via the special energetic link between this centre and the brow. Here, of course, it meets with mind which then attempts to understand it.

Psychic awareness enables us to be aware of subtle energetic phenomena, such as the light of the energy field around someone. It is the awareness that tells us, when we enter a room for example, that people have just had a row there. We actually pick up the vibrations of this happening before we even see their faces. The fabric of any building absorbs energy so that this faculty enables a sensitive person to be aware of past events that have happened in a place. These energies are external to us.

On the other hand, *intuitive awareness* enables us to be aware of messages from the Higher Self, and information from the spiritual levels – energies that are internal.

Our problem with all of the inputs to and from the brow centre is that once they are conveyed to the brain for interpretation, the mind steps in to act as uninvited consultant. But it is only able to compare information received with what it already knows and understands. If mind cannot match the information with our perceived life experience, it tends to put it straight in the reject tray.

Consciously or unconsciously, we have all had plenty of fun and games with our brow centre. Since ancient times it has been represented as, and called, the Third Eye because a way of seeing beyond the ordinary or the appearance of things seemed to originate here. This is exactly what it can do, in terms of both our psychic and intuitive awareness. Indeed, life is enhanced when we learn to use and trust these natural abilities. This is its challenge. For Distant Healers, the brow centre is the intuitive link with our Higher Self during attunement, as well as with the Higher Self of the person we are later working with.

The balanced centre vibrates to a deep royal blue or indigo light.

The crown centre

Located at the crown of the head, this centre is our link with the Source and provides a spiritual link with all other beings of Light. It deals with all issues of our spirituality and challenges us to acknowledge the spiritual truth of being and to allow this to be fully expressed in our lives.

The crown centre links with the body via the pineal gland. This gland tells us about the amount of sunlight we are getting and whether we are getting enough. It also mirrors the crown centre's role of telling us about the amount of spiritual Light we are allowing into our life – and whether this is enough. When we do not get enough sunlight, as those who live in 'grey' climates well know, we feel depressed. If deprivation goes on long enough, this can become the medical condition known as 'seasonal affective disorder' or 'SAD syndrome'. The remedy is to get some sunlight as soon as possible.

Deep depression or despair is very often a symptom of spiritual lack. This is why many cultures see such states as a disease of the spirit that should be tackled immediately. The remedy, of course, is a good dose of spiritual Light (which may not be the same thing as something religious).

The special energetic link with the base centre tells us that life is not about being either spiritual *or* human, but both. Life is a spiritual event and we, and all other beings, are an expression of the divine. The indigenous Lakota (or Sioux) people of North America proclaim this, during any sacred act or ceremony, when they pray: *Mitákuye oyásin! (*We are all related!) When we are living this expression of Oneness, the crown centre vibrates to the colour violet.

The human rainbow

Thus, at a subtle level, we are walking rainbows. All the colours are needed to make a rainbow, and this tells us that our life is, and always was, a complete whole. There is no issue or experience that does not have a valid place in our unique story. With this in mind, it is helpful to recall the functions of the seven main centres in relation to our total being. The lower three centres, via the mind, exert a pressure on the personality to engage in humanness.

The personality may well, and often does, interpret this to mean that this is all there is. The mind then tells us that there is plenty of logical and scientific argument to support this view. The upper three centres of the crown, brow and throat, via our intuition and feelings, exert a pressure on the personality to recall our light, or spiritual, origins.

The heart centre shows us that we will only ever be half of what we could be until we make the leap of faith and trust in our reality as soul. Through its processing of love issues, the heart centre shows us that love is the key to a harmonious balance of both aspects of our being. This is the message of all seven levels of consciousness, especially the crown and heart.

The centres of the hands and feet

Two further sets of subtle energy centres help us to keep our links with planet Earth, with the 'heavens' and with the expression of love that joins these two sacred aspects of being. The sole of the foot and palm centres link the polarity of the planetary energies with the two etheric polarity channels. In healing, these are accessed via the soles of the feet and the tops of the arms.

Linking energetically with the base centre, the centres in the soles of the feet absorb energies from the Earth (see Figure 15, on page 82). These life-giving energies are essential to the physical body and physical life. This is why it is good to go barefoot on the ground whenever you can, a practice that will lead to the pleasure of sensing the Earth in a deeper way. The soles of the feet act as grounding or earthing points, as does the base centre, for incoming subtle energies.

In the subtle sciences of Qi Gong and acupuncture, the *yongquan* point on the sole of the foot is connected to the kidneys and is a focus for treatment in cases of hypertension. This meridian point is in the same place as the sole of the foot centre (just behind the centre of the two large pads at the front of the foot) and its function gives a clue to the link between the centres of the feet and the base (since the base centre energies enter the body via the adrenal glands). Let's see what you can sense with your foot centres.

EXERCISE 26

Sensing Earth energies with the Sole-of-the-Foot Centres

- Stand on the ground with bare feet apart in relaxed posture. Take six slow breaths into the abdomen to attune yourself. Breathe normally.

- Put your mind in the soles of your feet. Be aware of your contact with the Earth, and the grass, soil, sand or whatever is under your feet. Close your eyes and notice whether you can sense an energetic transaction via the soles of your feet.

- Still with your focus in the feet, use the in-breath to aid your awareness of the passage of energy from the ground into your feet, up your legs to the base centre. Inhale a few times with this intention.

exercise continues ▶

- Note your discoveries. Repeat the exercise in different locations and at different times of the day. Again, what did you discover?

In Qi Gong the *laogong* point on the palm of the hand is related to the heart, blood circulation and to the release of negative *qi*, or heavy energy. This clue tells us about the vital energetic link between the palm centres and the heart (Figure 15, page 82). The link means that the palms of each hand can act as extensions of the heart in conveying love and healing. Hence we soothe, touch and caress with the hands. When the hands are used to hurt another there is a negative effect on the heart centre. Try the next exercise to see if you can sense the hand-heart link.

EXERCISE 27
Sensing the hand-heart energy circuit

This exercise extends the sensitivity you discovered and activated in the exercises so far. The first part focuses on drawing in energy, the second on giving it out.

- Sit in a relaxed position with the legs uncrossed. Hold your palms out in front of you with your arms bent at the elbow. Relax your elbows, the back of the neck and the shoulders. Close your eyes if this helps your concentration. Breathe normally.

- Focus your attention on the palm centres. As you inhale, sense that you can draw energy in through the centres. Breathe out gently, through the palms. Note your sensations.

- Now visualise the energetic link between your palms and your heart centre. Breathe in and sense energy moving up your arms, across your shoulders, to converge in the heart centre, in the middle of your chest.

exercise continues ▶

- Lower your arms and relax for a few moments. Raise your arms again, with your hands held out in front of you as before. In this second part of the exercise you are going to send energy from the heart centre to the palms.

- Focus on the heart centre and relax. Breathe into the heart centre. As you exhale, visualise energy moving from the heart centre, out to the shoulders, down the arms, to the centre in each palm. What did you sense this time?

- Compare your experiences of absorbing and transmitting energy via the palm and heart centres.

The experiences with the last two exercises reinforce your understanding of the role of the hands and feet in Distant Healing. The sole centres, through their contact with the planet, keep us grounded energetically and 'earth' energetic activity. This is important for our efficient functioning as a channel for healing energies, especially in the advanced out-of-body work we will be coming to shortly (see Chapter 10, page 113). Through the palm centres we transmit healing energies and we absorb energetic information. During this activity, the centres act like a kind of subtle eye.

We have a way of keeping in touch with the 'heavenly' realms, apart from via the crown centre. Our hands may hang at our sides for much of the time, but we can extend them in the opposite direction above our head. By holding the palm centres upwards, we can visualise breathing in the energies of the sun, sky and cosmos. This stance is a natural expression of joy and can be taken up to bring positive feelings and combat depression.

An issue for most individual Distant Healers, which also features on the agenda of most Distant Healing groups, is how to confront the feelings that surface during the work. These can arise when the request for help is made, when compiling the working list, even during the session itself. We also need to add to this the effects of information and life events on us.

The Distant Healing method presented here provides positive ways of addressing the subject and how to acquire these important skills is what we shall look at next.

Chapter 9

Addressing the effects of personal feelings and negative energies

Feelings and attunement

In my workshops on Distant Healing a recurring subject is whether it is appropriate for us to have feelings about our work. This question is inevitably countered with the assertion that the attunement process should be enough to keep us totally focused – personal feelings shouldn't come into it. My response is that both aspects of the work are true for most people. The attunement exercise in Chapter 1, page 17 is designed to align us with the Source of healing energies, but the link between attunement and feelings is highly relevant for us. So I am going to describe the process of addressing these points, using a combination of different responses from a number of typical workshop situations.

Whenever you practise any exercise it is within the context of what is happening around you and within you. The process of attunement challenges you to be aware of your inner state because your remaining in the heart centre depends on it. In honouring the attunement process, questions arise such as: What emotional energies are you bringing with you? Are you calm and untroubled? Or are you so unsettled by news or information recently received that conscious breathing and relaxation can only partially balance your emotional state?

Perhaps you are quite serene and looking forward to the work until you come to read your list. Then, without warning, a particular case creates a feeling that catches you off guard. Or, having become comfortably settled within your regular group meeting, you are upset when another member suddenly bursts into tears. Are you still focused or has your attention moved to the solar plexus centre? In other words, where are you?

Which brings us to the first and recurring problem: Is it all right to have feelings? On the positive side, we probably wouldn't want to do Distant Healing if we didn't care about others and the state of the world around us. This heartfelt feeling fuels positive motivation, energising us to act. On the negative side, the world is bombarding us with information, from far away and closer to home. Because we are sensitive, caring people, we are affected by this information, especially when it is some kind of disturbing or intimidating news.

Group experiences

At one workshop the group was asked how they would respond to a common anxiety: Should I go to the meeting this evening when I'm feeling so churned up; won't that affect the work of the group? And if I tell them why I'm churned up then everyone will be affected. Questions like these help the whole group. They press emotional buttons, and in this case some members felt threatened. They preferred to feel in control and unaffected rather than admit the possibility that a news happening, injury to a loved one, or a death in the family, could upset their equilibrium. Spirituality was about equanimity and control of the emotions.

We could have continued to discuss this, swinging back and forth between differing points of view. Instead I asked the group to listen to a two-minute tape of some real, though harrowing, radio news items. Every item had happened somewhere in the world within the past week. After a short pause, I asked if anyone would like to share how they were feeling after hearing the tape.

A young woman of 19 hung her head and sighed. 'I'm afraid of the world … because there's nothing I can do about it … Some days, I'm even afraid of being alive …' The man sitting next to her nodded. He understood because he was aware that he had had no education on how to deal with any form of negativity, and was filled with feelings which ranged from despair that he could do nothing to anger at his own helplessness.

There was some nervous moving about in seats, but by owning her feelings, the youngest member of the group had given everyone else permission to do the same. As others spoke up, it was soon obvious that the group felt an overwhelming sense of negativity and powerlessness. For some, this brought feelings of anger and despair.

Others had needed to tune out and simply ignore what they were hearing: 'This is what you hear every day. You have to find a way to cope with it or you'd be suicidal.'

'Turn it off – I turn it off! You don't have to listen to it.'

I switched the focus to how they felt in their bodies. Some said they sensed uncomfortable feelings in the solar plexus centre – sensations of pulling, churning, pain, burning, and attempts to close down feeling. Sensations in the heart centre were just as unpleasant – pulling, shrinking, squeezing, compression as if by a heavy weight, fogginess, loss of clarity and a closing down of love.

Finding a constructive strategy

When we are honest with ourselves we can at least admit that our emotional reactions to the media and other information affect our ability to work whole-heartedly as Distant Healers, and it is obvious that we need a strategy that is more constructive than mere coping. I asked the group to engage with finding a solution that evolved from this awareness. Most of us had stopped reading newspapers and some refused to listen to the news either on radio or TV. But when we considered this, the group reluctantly agreed that, as healers, we should not cut ourselves off from what was happening around us, or from happenings in the rest of the world. How could we send healing help if we weren't aware of all that was going on? The other position was that these were good reasons for sticking to the 'list' and working solely with requests for help. But again, the majority felt that this was a kind of short-sightedness at best, or an ostrich-like response at worst. Our times demanded that we look further than the list. We knew that positive thought can affect situations, how much more good could be done with Distant Healing. This brought us back to the need for a strategy that kept us in touch with news events, while encouraging us to work with them.

How the 'list' affects us

At this point I suggested we should first look at whether simply sticking to the list really did shield us from feelings. To test this, we listened carefully as each of us read out our lists. Then I asked group members to describe their feelings on reading their own list and on hearing the lists of the rest of the group. First there came the urge and desire to help, a welling up of love in the heart centre. There was a pause as we contemplated these fine feelings. Then, one by one, members owned up to feelings of guilt, anger, resentment, tiredness, grief and wanting to cry. Some confessed to letting their minds wander and realised this was a tuning-out strategy.

Initially, the group members were shocked by their own revelations. Distant Healing was an act of unconditional love. Why hadn't attunement kept them in the place of compassion? They looked around the circle at each other. There were long faces, sad faces and bewildered faces.

Then suddenly there was a burst of laughter. 'Look at us. We're so disappointed that we're not saints!' This remark broke the tension and there was more laughter.

'I admit it,' said a would-be saint. 'Sometimes I'm really affected just hearing myself reading out my list. Then tonight it happened again hearing someone else's list – realising that each one of them was in trouble or was trying to deal with some problem.' This brought tears to quite a few eyes.

The learning from all this is that we are deeply affected by the daily doses of negativity that come our way and also by the unending healing challenge they represent. A similar emotional challenge is presented by our encountering requests for help, and then dealing with these requests. These emotional impacts affect us whether we choose to work solo or with a group.

The two energetic situations

Two energetic situations emerge from our findings. In the first situation, the emotions that we generate *within* ourselves, for whatever reason, affect our energy centres, the endocrine glands and the physical body. Their impact will be 'positive' or 'negative', as I explain below.

Secondly, information coming from outside us carries an actual energy. Energies like this also impact on the centres and the physical body. In this second scenario, for our purposes I will only describe what happens when the energy of *negative* news and information impacts on us.

Both of these energetic processes begin in the solar plexus centre, and they may happen separately or in tandem. Towards the end of this chapter there are three exercises which combine to deal positively with these processes. This positive coping strategy will help you to address energetic impacts, as well as your feelings and reactions.

Situation 1: How our emotions affect the centres and glands

Emotions are first processed in the solar plexus centre, the centre linked to the mind and its messages. Any message received by this centre activates the brow centre. You recall that one of the tasks of this centre is to pass intuitive or soul knowledge to us so that we can compare this with the mind's conditioned information. However, most people have a problem with accepting their intuitive wisdom. This activity goes on to affect different endocrine glands in the physical, producing a range of possible physical conditions.

If the solar plexus centre receives a 'positive' (life-enhancing, compatible or loving) message, the brow centre signals this to its 'light' link with the pineal gland. This then triggers the thymus gland to strengthen the immune system which, in turn, has a very positive effect on the heart centre. These energetic activities explain how emotions influence the body, but they also explain how positive thinking and positive attitudes bring harmony, peace and health to the system.

What happens, then, if the reverse takes place? If the solar plexus centre receives a 'negative' (life-denying, incompatible or loveless) message, in order to protect the route to the pineal and the gland itself, the brow centre closes, preventing energetic flow. The pineal gland is not just sensitive to the amount of light in our physical environment, but is sensitive to the amount of spiritual Light in our energetic environment. The effect of brow centre closure on the pineal is that it creates pressure for more light.

This only reinforces the closing of the brow. The unbalanced state of the pineal gland adversely affects the thymus gland, so that the immune system is also under threat and does not function efficiently. These energetic activities explain how trauma, negative emotional experiences, as well as negative attitudes, influence the body, especially undermining its ability to fight off disease.

You are beginning to build up a picture of health outcomes that are the result of your emotional life. This adds to your essential knowledge base, and you can apply this knowledge to yourself so that you remain healthy and able to do your healing work. Before you can do this, you also have to understand that everything in life is radiating energy, and that you need to be particularly aware of those energies that are moving towards you. These include the negative energies of news and information.

Situation 2: How negative information energy affects the centres

The energetic impact of *negative news, signals and information* creates a second, often parallel, response which is just as damaging as that caused by our emotional reactions. In this case we are looking at the impact of massive doses of negative energy on all the energy centres: these reactions will be taking place irrespective of our emotional response.

Our leaders, and those in positions of responsibility, probably do not realise what is happening to their citizens and, if they did, they would have no idea how to deal with the problem. We must find our own way to deal with the impact on our personal world, and the effects on our energy centres.

The mind is the first part of us to absorb the negative energy of a message, whether from the media, a letter, a telephone message or a conversation. We feel the immediate impact as a threat to our sense of safety and security. This is because of the process outlined as follows.

The mind cues the solar plexus centre to receive the energies. Their negative quality is interpreted as a threat which triggers the defensive emotion of fear. This, in turn, generates the energies of stress and anxiety. These stresses impact on the person's sense of self, their sense of personal power and self-worth. At the same time the digestive system and nearby organs are affected via the endocrine glands in the pancreas.

The overall threat is to personal survival so that the negative energy is pulled down towards the base centre, via the sacral. Here it begins to undermine the expression of joy, creativity and sexuality. The lower abdomen and lower back are affected via the sex glands.

From there it moves to the base centre where it undermines our sense of personal survival, encouraging detachment from the natural world, fear of natural processes, fear of ageing, even fear of death. As the energies impact on the lower body and legs, via the adrenal glands, they also affect the consciousness of each cell in the body.

Because of the link between the base and heart centres, the energetic impact of negativity next moves there. The organs of the chest are affected, via the thymus gland. We develop a sense that there is no longer love, compassion or justice in the world.

The energies continue moving upwards to the throat centre. The organs of the ear, nose and throat are affected, via the thyroid gland. The subtle effect is that we feel we have no voice, we are not heard, and we cannot be who we really are. Instead we become more concerned about how we appear to others. There is a lack of trust as truth seems to become devalued.

The brow centre is next affected. The physical impact, via the pituitary gland and the hypothalamus, is on the head, eyes and brain. But the pituitary also oversees all other glands and their production of hormones. When the brow centre is undermined, we lose trust in our own intuition. This means that we lose our connection with knowing what is right for us and what is not.

Instead, we feel the need to put more reliance on the thoughts and opinions of others. We tend to take less responsibility for our acts and choices, and look to a leader, or even some sort of messianic figure, to solve our problems. The brow centre tries to assure us that nothing is solved outside of us, but we are already having a problem listening to and heeding our intuitive self.

Our crown centre finally receives the negative energetic messages. A range of spiritual and existential problems join with the mental and emotional turmoil that incessant doses of negativity create. This centre processes all issues about our link with the Source and the Light of the Source. We wonder if we can ever make contact with the Source within, even if it did in fact exist. The physical effects on the pineal gland are similar to those described in the previous section on the route of emotional energy.

The world has an impact on every energy centre

In this way, the world is impacting on every centre, and, through them, the physical body. The first signs that we, or our body, are trying to cope with high doses of negativity are the appearance of any of the symptoms described above: stress, anxiety, tiredness and the early stages of bodily disease.

But we should always remember that the body is our friend. It is designed and formed for life, even when some life events may be destructive. We are genetically endowed with the ability to withstand a certain level of negative effects. We can recall that life is for the manifestation of the divine Source, our true reality.

Our friend the body has various ways of warning us when the limits of tolerance have been reached. We should listen and take heed and be aware firstly, that mind will often try to override bodily messages. Secondly, when the body is calling to us, problems may already be manifesting on the mental and emotional levels. The way that we deal with negative energies will determine whether they have the power to nullify the life-affirming, life-building, health-creating energies of our own being.

A way of ensuring our health and safety is through the threefold empowerment strategy of accepting our feelings.

Accepting the message of our feelings

The heart centre is the balancing and harmonising point in the system. At the same time it is the centre that processes all issues concerned with love. It is where we find our response to lovelessness. This is the place where we attune to the Source, where our mental intention is given its soul dimension and from where the energies of healing emanate.

This is why the impact of emotions is so important in our work. Feelings and emotions are not good or bad, right or wrong, in themselves. They carry no judgement or moral overtone. We should, however, listen to our feelings because they are the language the Higher Self uses to indicate whether something is appropriate for us or not. Our level of discomfort acts as a scale we can use to help us decide about this.

A common feeling of discomfort occurs when feelings are not expressed. A lump in the throat, pain, burning, or a feeling of blockage there, all signal that some feeling is not being expressed and should be. When things in our life are not true, or not being expressed when they need to be, the throat centre responds. This discomfort extends to things such as not being creative or not doing what we feel we want to do in life. Sometimes we block our positive expressions of love and joy. We may even find that our own inhibitions urge us to block others' positive expressions.

Missing the real message

Returning to the Distant Healing Circle, this is exactly what can happen here. It is possible to misinterpret the impact of positive energies, on us or someone else, especially when the mind interprets this according to its own conditioning. I was working with a group when a woman collapsed sobbing. Members who had never encountered this wondered if something had gone wrong. They wondered too why I did not jump up and pass her the box of tissues. This woman was later able to explain to the group how the influx of healing energy, with its powerful feelings of love and beauty, completely overwhelmed her. She was crying with joy!

This can happen to an individual whether working solo or in a group. It is not an emotion but a reaction to the energy of love. At such times it is not a loving gesture to block the person's reactions by offering reassurance such as tissues or a pat on the back. The best reassurance is the silent, loving support of sitting with them, being there for them. People must be allowed to express what is happening within. It was an important experience for the group to learn to accept what can happen.

Body awareness and energetic flow

Feelings, then, need to be welcomed. This is because they are expressions of energetic happenings and energy needs to flow. Energetic flow allows the system to rebalance itself and return to harmony. An interruption to this process, no matter how well meant, creates an energy block. This is the key to the next three exercises which are designed to help you address your feelings by permitting their energetic flow. We begin by becoming more deeply aware of our body.

EXERCISE 28
Body awareness

- Sit or lie comfortably. Use the breath to relax your body and allow your breathing to settle to a gentle rhythm.

- As you link with the rhythm of your breath, visualise that your body is surrounded by a sphere of golden light. Notice how you become calm and serene as your awareness of the normally peaceful operations within your body increases.

- Take a moment to remind yourself that this is the vehicle for your soul's expression on Earth. Your consciousness helped to make it what it is today. You dwell within this body where a million movements of energy are continually taking place. You can join the smallest or the greatest part of this activity through your link with the body consciousness.

- Gently scan round your body. Notice where your attention is drawn to first. Try to maintain this relaxed attention as you continue to scan round your body.

- You are sitting or lying on something. Notice what this feels like. Notice what you sense, what you hear.

- Become aware of your breathing again and notice any feelings of discomfort. Without trying to interpret them, pay attention to these bodily sensations.

- As you relax into the light that surrounds you, allow yourself to be. Mentally affirm: 'I am.'

That exercise can be continued for as long as you wish, but it should be for not less than five minutes. As a simple tool for being with your body, it is another building block of Distant Healing.

EXERCISE 29
Accessing body secrets

- In the same position as above, relax and breathe normally. Recall that the operations of the body are based in the cells. Because of energetic and cellular consciousness, the body is able to store memories about anything that has happened to it from the time of conception until now.

- Allow your attention to focus on the first body part that comes to mind (don't think about it). Allow this part to show you what it has stored. Accept what comes without judgement or self-judgement. It may be in the form of pictures, words or sensations.

If you have been ill or have suffered an injury, listen to what your body may have to tell you about it. If you locate a certain mood or feeling somewhere in your body, allow these parts of yourself to talk to you about your perceptions and sensations. By allowing your body to draw your attention to a certain part, your intuition comes into play. This part is speaking to you because it is the right moment to communicate what it has to say and for you to pay attention to this.

When communication has finished, in your mind's eyes see the golden glow of energy around you change to pink, the colour of love. Allow this pink light to penetrate every part of your body. Give thanks for this light and its effects.

Working with your feelings: from coping to empowerment

In the two previous exercises, you had the opportunity to become aware of how feelings find a place in the body. Having got used to how your body communicates this, you can further develop the relationship by addressing the issue we have been looking at – how to own our powerful feelings, and the impact of negative energies on the system, in a positive and constructive way. The next exercise completes the empowerment strategy.

The first stage of the exercise is acknowledging that feelings and reactions arise in us. They originate in the subtle energy system and are not simply created in the mind as fearful imaginings. Then recognise that they are energies and that this kind of energy should be kept moving, allowed to flow. The second stage is acceptance of your feelings and acceptance of energetic impacts. This allows energetic flow. Once you can allow and encourage the flow of your own, as well as incoming energies, you will find that your system can return you to a state of balance. Resistance works against this innate ability. Since we were children, we have learned to block energy flow, but as Distant Healers we now have to learn how to remove these blocks.

EXERCISE 30
Working with your feelings

- Make sure that you will not be disturbed during this exercise. Sit or lie comfortably alone. It is not necessary to relax the body or do anything that will calm your feelings.

- Begin by focusing on how you are feeling. Don't worry about your breathing or relaxation. Notice your thoughts, and what is going on in your body, as you pay attention to your feelings.

- Increase your awareness of your feelings by deciding why you feel happy; or why you feel uncomfortable; or why you feel frightened; or why you feel sad; and so on.

- Notice whether you tend to judge yourself. Notice whether you offer resistance to the exercise. Try to just observe and no more.

- Now deepen your experience of your feelings by simply accepting them unconditionally. Just as they are, right now. Relax into this acceptance. These are your feelings.

exercise continues ▶

- As you become aware of your breathing, breathe with the feelings as if you are aligning with them and flowing with them. Breathe your feelings.

- Now, as you gently take time, your breath and your feelings gradually come to a place of balance. Take your time. Stay with what you are now feeling.

- Bring your attention to your heart centre, consciously opening it, as if you are opening the 'arms' of your heart. Welcome the balance of feelings into your heart centre.

- Become aware of your whole being in a state of peace. Stay in this peace-filled awareness.

By really becoming aware of your feelings, by identifying them, by accepting and experiencing them, you allow their impact on you, and your reactions to them, to be released into healing. By practising this exercise you will come to understand what feelings and emotions are. You are not your emotions. You realise that your emotions need not control you.

Where they produce fearful reactions in the solar plexus centre, with the previous exercise you *consciously* move the energies up into your heart centre (instead of the unconscious movement down into the sacral centre as described earlier). You are consciously moving the energy flow to the place of balance and unconditional love. Again, if you practise this exercise with a partner or a group, you will gain great benefits through sharing your experiences. The group energy also enhances the constructive process of the exercise.

In the case of your strong reaction to the flow of healing energies through you, through the group, or from another in your group, carry out the same procedure. Notice whether you are still in your heart centre or if your reactions, or the reactions of others, have moved the flow down to your solar plexus centre.

Feelings are an important part of your energetic makeup. They are a reminder of who you are – essentially a being of love. We all need to express love and receive love. Positive feelings are a natural expression of love. Negative feelings are a natural response to lovelessness. The personal challenge is not to add to the energies of lovelessness by word, thought or deed, thereby closing down the system against love, but to return to the heart centre. This is the challenge to Distant Healers with every call for help that they receive.

Having begun to study the energetic impact of living in the world, of absorbing negative energies, of confronting healing issues, or even the effect of Love itself, you are better equipped to add some more advanced techniques to your way of working. Some of these may take you out of your physical body, which may sound strange, but is actually quite natural. You move 'out of your body' every night when you go to sleep, something you have been doing since you were in the womb!

Chapter 10

Advanced distant healing

Multi-dimensional you

If we become enclosed in our own feelings, we soon feel separation from others and the world, even separation from the wonder of the multi-dimensional self described in Chapter 3, page 27. I emphasise that we can avoid this by returning to the heart centre, for here we are aligned with the source of multi-dimensional life. Here, we know that Distant Healing is possible because we are all One, united energetically as well as spiritually. Here, we know that energy follows thought because this is one of the laws of Love. Prayerful intention is a means of crossing all dimensions, travelling to the source of Creation, instantly, because that Source is actually within each of us, closer than breathing.

You know that you have a physical reality, an emotional reality, and a mental reality. Distant Healing is now going to introduce you to another aspect of our total spiritual reality. We are conscious of our body, our thoughts and feelings, from time to time our dreams, plus all the sensory information that we take in from the world around us.

But the possibility of being conscious of other levels is always there. So as well as sending out our healing intentions from our solo or group base, it is possible for us to make another kind of contact with those subjects that are at a distance from us. We may be aware of this contact with our everyday consciousness or not. This usually depends on two factors: how necessary conscious contact is, and our mental, intuitive and spiritual development.

Life outside of the physical Body

At the end of the last chapter, I mentioned how you have out-of-body experiences on a regular basis when you sleep. This is possible because the spiritual you, the Higher Self, is the real you. You were a reality before your body came into existence and you will exist after your body ceases to be. You can, and do, detach yourself from the physical, with its etheric bridging level, to travel outside the space-time continuum. This enables you to do a range of things which you could not do when confined to your physical body.

You can, for example, meet up with those who teach you; you can make contact with those who have passed over (so that everyone actually gets proof, during their own lifetime, that consciousness continues after physical death). Your mind then tries to make sense of this information and, more often than not, presents it to you as a 'dream'.

When these dream experiences are not simply a means of sorting out what has been going on in your mind (such as the happenings of that day), they are probably the out-of-body experiences I referred to. When your dream experience is vivid, unforgettable, and in colour, it is a message from your Higher Self. You need to take time to absorb such messages. Your intuition will guide you, not the mind. The mind will only be able to compare it with previous data already stored. A better use of mind is to record such activities in order to enhance everyday living and your life journey.

The other important thing that happens to you is that you use the sleep state to travel out of your body to help and heal those in need. Again, your mind tries to make sense of that 'dream' too. The whole realm of healing in the sleep state is fascinating, not least because you can be doing it, but you are not conscious of it. In other words, the information is not transferred to your everyday awareness. Nevertheless, this is another aspect of Distant Healing.

I frequently receive telephone calls, letters and emails from all over the world, thanking me for appearing to somebody to help them. In most of these cases I have no recollection of the encounter whatsoever and they may not even be on my Distant Healing list!

These things are part of my experience, but you may feel the need for explanations. The pioneering work of physicists and mathematicians, such as Professor William A. Tiller, has done much to provide a scientific rationale for the phenomenon of out-of-body experiences. A very clear account of his work, as it applies to Distant Healing, appears in Dr Richard Gerber's *Vibrational Medicine* (see references to both researchers in Further Reading and Web Resources, pages 196 and 200).

The astral level, astral travelling and Distant Healing

The phenomenon of travelling outside the physical body has always been known. In Western cultures it came to be called *astral travelling*, derived from the Latin and Ancient Greek for 'star' (*astrum/astron*). We sleep when the stars appear, hence 'astral travelling' came to mean travelling in the sleep state, in your astral body, on the astral level. This so-called astral level is simply any level of being outside the physical, when you are in your astral body – which can happen at any time, not just when asleep. Being 'out of body' is being in your astral body.

The astral body has a frequency band which at its lowest range lies between the etheric and the emotional energy zones.

Like the physical body, the astral body has energetic links to the etheric, emotional, mental and soul energy zones. The subtle energy system pervades all these zones, and the energetic activity within them is conveyed to and from them via the energy centres.

Some healers are able to move on to the astral level to carry out Distant Healing during their waking state. This may be a conscious or unconscious experience. So people may describe how the healer appeared to them, yet the healer has no waking knowledge of this.

In Distant Healing, energetic tracks or pathways are opened up so that conscious astral level healing can occur in two basic ways. You either find that you can 'travel' (in your astral body) to the person needing help or the person is 'brought' to you in *their* astral body. Some Distant Healers like to work this way, especially when there is an emergency call for their help. It is quite possible to train yourself to travel in your astral body, but most healers have not reached this state of conscious control over their astral movements and are happy to rely on soul guidance as to when and how the travelling will take place. I advise that you assume this attitude and go with the flow of soul too.

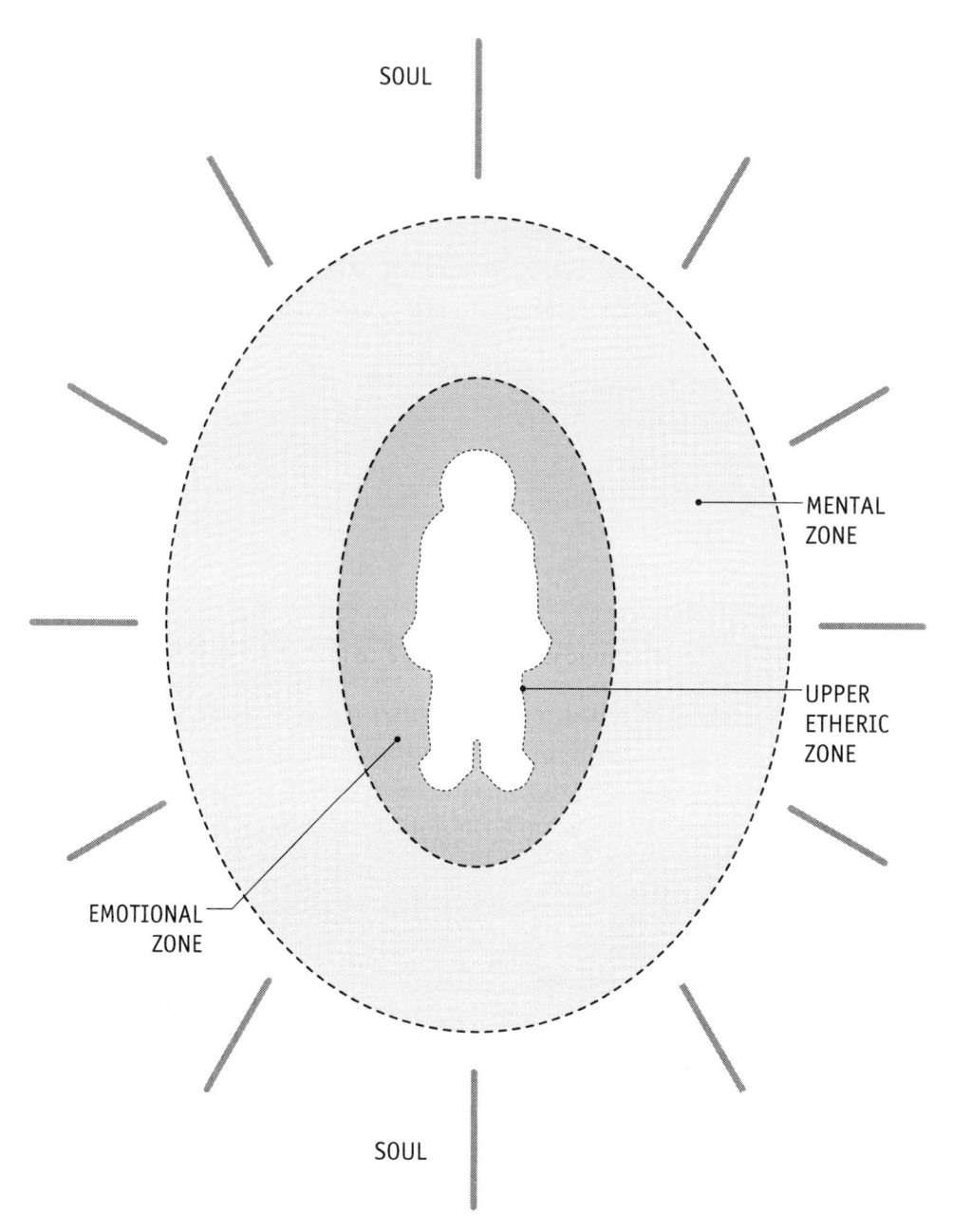

Figure 19. The energy field of the astral body

In Distant Healing, keep it simple and natural at all times. The astral level exercises, like all the exercises here, should only be used for the healing purposes specified.

Astral level healing

The next exercise is designed to help you begin conscious astral level healing, if you are guided, or inspired, to work this way. I describe it as an advanced way of working, but it is a natural development of Distant Healing and your own development as a Distant Healer. Practise it a number of times and keep a record of what you experience. This will enable you to assess which way you tend to work and which feels most comfortable for you.

If you have any queries about the exercise, get your working partner to join you as a passive observer and supporter. In the Introduction I described how, when I got back from Italy, I soon found myself doing astral level healing without even trying; it was the most natural way for me to work.

EXERCISE 31

Astral level healing

Though you always work with the subject, rather than the condition, in astral level work you will often be aware of your hands moving into the area of a stated condition, as well as other important sites such as the centres. Go with the flow of your guidance and make a note of what happens later.

- Make sure that you will not be interrupted in any way. Prepare and dedicate your working space. Have your list of subjects to hand. Attune yourself, light your candle and dedicate the work. Ask to be used as a channel for healing, and to be guided by your Higher Self (soul). You will look forward to being directed by this source (whether or not you will be doing any Distant Healing at the astral level).

- Sit with your feet flat on the floor with your hands, palms up, on your thighs or in your lap. The hands should not overlap or touch. (In astral work it is essential for the palm centres to remain active,

exercise continues ▶

hence the palms-up position of the hands.) Use the breath to calm and relax the body. Let go of any worries or anxieties with the out-breath, through the open mouth. When you feel attuned, close your mouth and breathe normally. Check that your body is relaxed, including the back of the neck, the shoulders and pelvis. Sit in the silence for a few moments.

- Now take the first request on your list. Mention the subject by name because the vibration of the name strengthens your link with them (as in the Healing Triangle, see Figure 1, page 12).

- Close your eyes to aid concentration and wait quietly and patiently to see if you become aware that the subject is in front of you.

- If you have been 'taken' to the person, or the person has been 'brought' to you, you will sense this. This becomes easier when you relax and accept that it is possible for this to happen. You will also be able to sense whether the adult person, child, or baby is lying or sitting in front of you and how the body is orientated.

- Mentally make sure that you are comfortably orientated to carry out what needs to be done. Allow your intuitive guidance to help you sense where your hands need to go.

- Let's take an example as illustration. Your help has been requested for a man who has problems with movement on the whole of the right side of his body. In this case, once you are aware of his astral body in front of you, you will probably feel drawn to hold your hands over the area in question: the right side of the body.

- If this is what he needs, you will feel healing energy leave your hands – or whatever sign tells you that you are working. Move down the rest of the right side as far as you find energy to be needed.

- Keep your hands over each area until you feel a change in the flow of energy, which could be sensed as a marked decrease, or falling off, in intensity. The signal is that all, or part, of the healing is complete.

exercise continues ▶

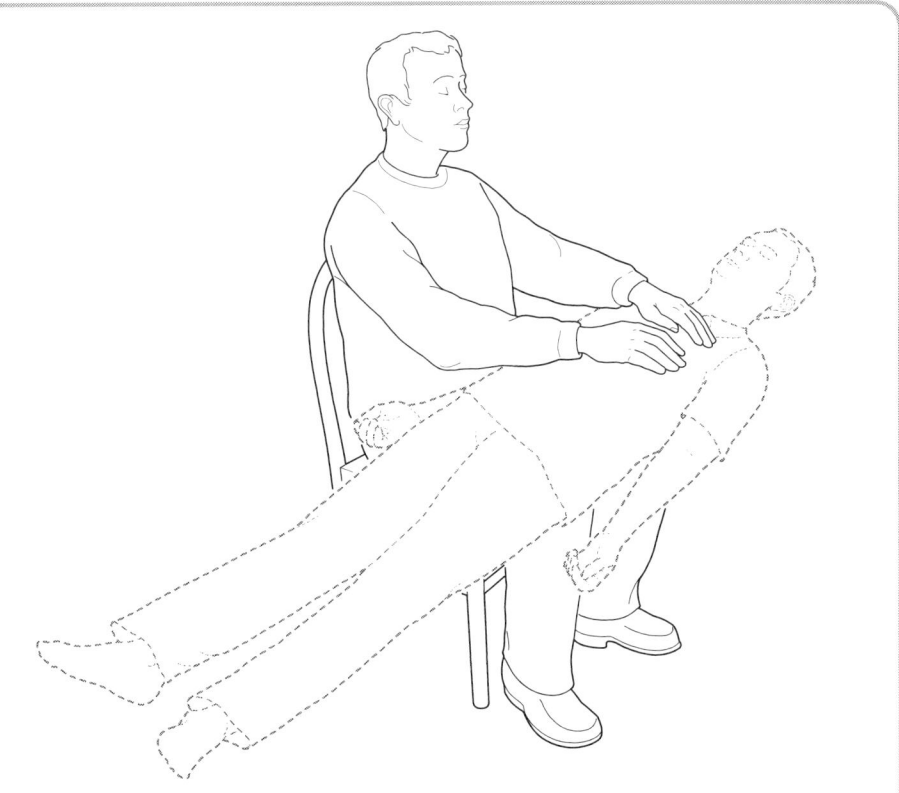

Figure 20. Astral level healing

- Wait for your guidance to see if you need to give healing elsewhere. There may be a centre involved, for example, or you may need to move your hands to somewhere other than the right side of the body.

- The energetic activity in your hands is confirmation that this is not taking place in your imagination. A person with developed perceptions would be able to sense or 'see' what was going on and confirm that you were working this way.

- When you have completed your work with that person, mentally thank them. Now take a full breath and, as you exhale, surround them with a protective sphere of light. This may be done mentally or by raising your arms and moving your hands gently to make a sphere around the astral body in front of you.

exercise continues ▶

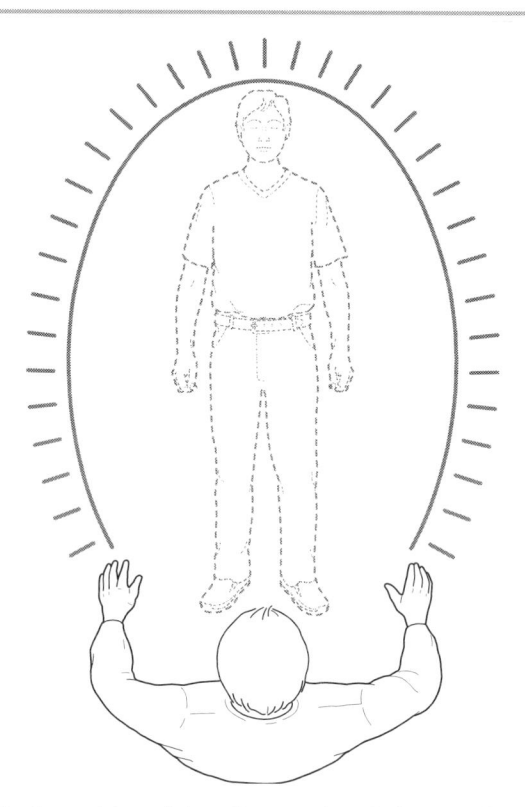

Figure 21. Astral level healing – the Sphere of Protection

- At this point, either the Distant Healing subject returns to their physical body, or you return to your physical body. You may also remain in the astral body state to receive the next subject on your list in the same way. Or you may both return to the physical state.

- If there is another subject to work with, first make sure that the one you were working on is no longer in front of you (they have returned to their physical). Now visualise clearing silver light washing over your upraised palms. You can now proceed to the next subject on your list. Take a short pause if you feel the need.

- Follow the same procedure as before. Finally break your link with the last subject by clearing your hands.

exercise continues ▶

- When you have completed your work, blow out the candle. This can be done by sending out the light of the candle. Pause for a moment and see if you intuitively feel where it needs to go. This is usually the first place that comes to mind. As you blow out the candle, say: 'I send the Light out to –.'

- Carry out the Closing-down Procedure outlined in Chapter 5, pages 56–7.

If, during an astral level healing, you sense that you are no longer sitting in your chair, but standing over or by the subject, this tells you that you have travelled to them. Keep relaxed and proceed as described above. You are quite safe and can move out of this state whenever you like.

This way of working is very satisfying. Even so, it requires intense, but relaxed concentration. Because of this, I recommend that you start astral level healing with one subject at a time, with an aim of no more than six in any one session, unless guided otherwise. You need to feel totally comfortable and build up your confidence so that you do not get tired by the level of focused effort needed to work this way.

Keep a note of what happens in your Healing journal and try to get some feedback about your work whenever possible.

Working together

It is good to compare notes with another or others who are working on the astral level. Networking gives you the opportunity to share and gain knowledge and insight from the experience of others. It acts as a form of peer supervision and helps to keep everyone's 'feet on the ground'. This can be done with your Distant Healing Circle, having the aim of working on the astral level. As before, you will need someone to lead or facilitate each time you meet, and every member should take a turn at this. In the following exercises, I suggest two basic ways of working.

EXERCISE 32

The astral level Healing Circle – with one joint list

Before working together, the whole of this exercise should be read to the group so that everyone is clear about how to proceed.

Make sure that you will not be disturbed and disconnect all telephones. Have a circle of chairs, in the centre of which is a candle that can be safely placed on the ground. The group should have one list which you have compiled together. The length of the list will be dictated by the time you have together, but should be no more than six to ten tasks, unless intuitively guided otherwise. The group agrees on one nominated member to carry out the work as outlined below.

- The group sits in a circle with feet flat on the floor and their hands, palms up, on their thighs or in their laps. The hands should not overlap or touch. The group leader should help the group to attune and follow these guidelines:

- 'Use the breath to calm and relax the body. Let go of any worries or anxieties with the out-breath, through the open mouth. Close the mouth, when you feel attuned, and breathe normally. Check that your body is relaxed, including the back of the neck, the shoulders and pelvis. Allow the calm silence to settle on our Circle.'

- The leader lights the candle and dedicates the light to the work of the Distant Healing Circle, asking for the protection and guidance of the Source of healing energies.

- 'Visualise the light of the candle as the light of these energies and breathe it in to the heart centre. Allow the light to fill your chest.'

- 'Now pass the energy in your heart centre to the person on your left, until you are all linked together.' Intuitively, you may have to wait to gather your heart energy before you can pass it on.

exercise continues ▶

- The leader should be aware of this and allow enough time for group linking, for this is the foundation of the healing circle. Most people will also sense when the circle is linked.

- The leader expresses the purpose of the meeting and gives thanks, on behalf of the group, for the opportunity to be of service. 'Focus on the Light in the heart centre. See this Light extending from you to the centre of the Circle. This builds a central column of Light: the Light of healing.'

- The leader announces the group's first task: 'We ask to be used as channels for healing for (the name of the person, animal, situation, etc. on the list).'

- The group waits for the subject to appear (to their inner vision) in the centre of the circle.

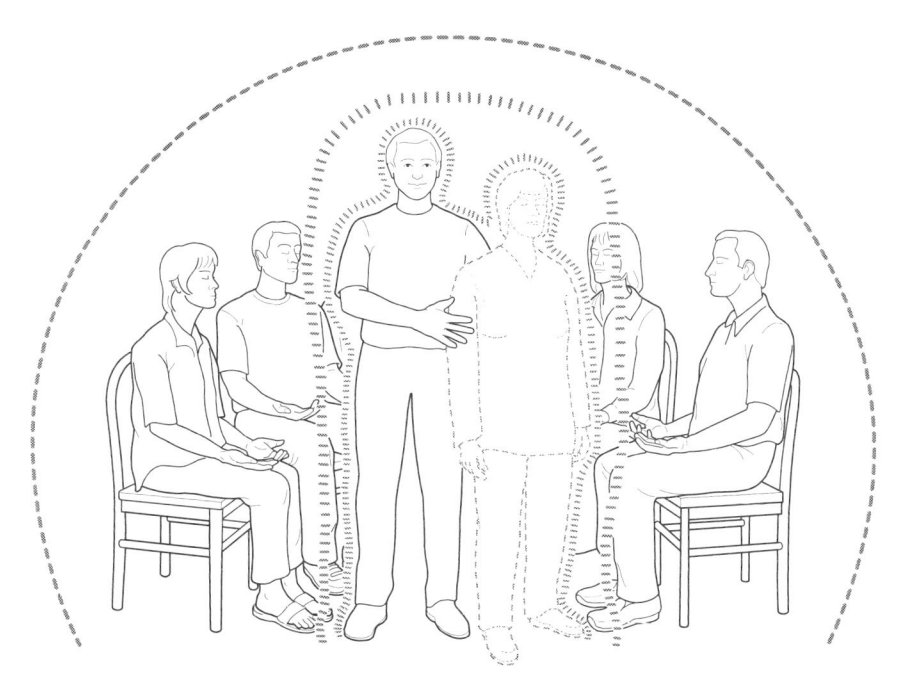

Figure 22. The astral level Healing Circle

exercise continues ▶

- As soon as the nominated member is aware of this, they begin work on the subject just as in Exercise 31, page 117. The rest of the group contributes to the healing by sitting in awareness, creating a powerful group energy which will be used in the healing work. At this stage, members may sense energy moving from their hands.

- Other group members may feel intuitively that they need to use their hands also. This should only occur once the nominated healer has begun to work.

- The leader monitors group activity. Work is completed on the first named subject when the healer has ceased hand activity and returned their hands to the resting position (palms down). The leader indicates this to the group with a gentle signal, such as a bell or with the words: 'We have completed the work for (name).' On hearing this, group members return their hands to the resting position.

- The leader then announces the next task and the group proceeds as before, with a different nominated healer each time.

- When the list is complete, the leader indicates this to the group. Sit together in the silence.

- The leader closes the Circle by expressing thanks, on behalf of the group, and by sending the light out to where it is needed. This is usually the first place that comes to mind.

- Every member of the group takes steps to become well grounded by rubbing their hands together and becoming aware of their feet in contact with the ground. The leader checks that everyone is grounded. The group can celebrate their heart-based work in whatever way seems appropriate.

- Discuss your work together. Share experiences and queries to consolidate learning. During this reflection session, allocate time to make notes, or illustrate the experience in some way. This allows the members to log their experience and learning, chart the energies

exercise continues ▶

they have been working with, and ground the experience. It also gives the mind time to absorb what has happened and for it to log the naturalness of this form of altered-state work.

The Circle could be followed by a group activity such as meditation, a reading, listening to music, etc. In the case of meditation, since it is a continuation of the same altered state of consciousness, it should take place *before* closing the Circle, as mentioned above. Afterwards, the leader sends out the light and makes sure everyone is grounded. Before the group disperses, carry out the Closing-down Procedure (pages 56–7) together.

The second basic astral level healing method is very much like the procedure for working solo, but instead you are working with the support and energy of the group.

EXERCISE 33

The astral level Healing Circle – with individual lists

Before working together, the whole of this exercise should be read to the group so that everyone is clear about how to proceed.

Make sure that you will not be disturbed and disconnect all telephones. Have a circle of chairs, in the centre of which is a candle that can be safely placed on the ground. Every member of the group should have their own list ready. The length of the list will be dictated by the time you have together, but should be no more than six to ten tasks, unless intuitively guided otherwise. The nominated group leader does not have a list, but monitors what is happening to every member and the Circle as a whole. Though you always work with the subject, rather than the condition, in astral level work you will often be aware of your hands moving into the area of a stated condition, as well as other important sites such as the centres.

exercise continues ▶

Go with the flow of your guidance and make a note of what happens later.

- The group sits in a circle with feet flat on the floor and their hands, palms up, on their thighs or in their laps. The hands should not overlap or touch. The leader helps the group to attune and follow these guidelines:

- 'Use the breath to calm and relax the body. Let go of any worries or anxieties with the out-breath, through the open mouth. Close the mouth, when you feel attuned, and breathe normally. Check that your body is relaxed, including the back of the neck, the shoulders and pelvis. Allow the calm silence to settle on the group.'

- The leader lights the candle and dedicates the light to the work of the Distant Healing Circle, asking for the protection and guidance of the Source of healing energies.

- 'Visualise the light of the candle as the Light of these energies and breathe it in to the heart centre. Allow the Light to fill your chest.'

- 'Now pass the energy in your heart centre to the person on your left, until you are all linked together.' Intuitively, you may have to wait to gather your heart energy before you can pass it on.

- The group leader should be aware of this and allow enough time for group linking, for this is the foundation of the Healing Circle. Most people will also sense when the Circle is linked.

- The leader expresses the purpose of the meeting and gives thanks, on behalf of the group, for the opportunity to be of service. 'Focus on the Light in the heart centre. See this Light extending from you to the centre of the Circle. This builds a central column of Light: the Light of healing.'

- The leader announces the group's task: 'We ask to be used as channels for healing for those we each name mentally.'

exercise continues ▶

- Each group member waits for their first subject to appear (to their inner vision) in front of them. As soon as they are aware of this, they begin work on the subject just as in the previous solo exercise, so that members are working simultaneously. Each member should take the time needed for the task. The whole group is also creating a powerful energy which will be used in each person's healing work.

- The leader monitors group activity, keeping an eye on the progress of the whole circle. In so doing, the leader also contributes to the group energy.

- Work is completed on the first named subject when you sense that hand activity has ceased. Return hands to the resting position (palms down).

- Take a few moments before choosing the next subject on your list. Work with them in the same way. When you have completed your list, return your hands to the resting position. Wait patiently for the leader to signal that everyone has completed their task list. Realise that you are still contributing to the group energy during this time.

- When every member of the group has reached the point of completion, the leader indicates this to the group with a gentle signal, such as a bell or with the words: 'We have completed our work. Let us sit together in the silence.'

- The leader closes the Circle by expressing thanks, on behalf of the group, and by sending the Light out to where it is needed. This is usually the first place that comes to mind.

- Every member takes steps to become well grounded by rubbing their hands together and becoming aware of their feet in contact with the ground. The leader checks that everyone is grounded. The group can celebrate their heart-based work in whatever way seems appropriate.

exercise continues ▶

- Discuss your work together. Share experiences and queries to consolidate learning. During this reflection session, allocate time to make notes, or illustrate the experience in some way. This allows the group members to log their experience and learning, chart the energies they have been working with, and ground the experience. It also gives the mind time to absorb what has happened, and for it to log the naturalness of this form of altered-state work.

The Circle could be followed by a group activity such as meditation, a reading, listening to music, etc. In the case of meditation, since it is a continuation of the same altered state of consciousness, it should take place *before* closing the Circle, as mentioned above. Afterwards, the leader sends out the Light and makes sure everyone is grounded. Before the group disperses, carry out the Closing-down Procedure (pages 56–7) together.

The two basic ways of astral level healing could be alternated. Or members may have a preference and the group can decide on a common way of working together.

Distant Healing and life issues

A common request for Distant Healing is to help the terminally ill to pass over, to help the bereaved who are left behind, or to help one who has already passed over. Families also ask for help when a baby is expected and the healing will be directed to the mother, the incoming soul, and to the obstetric and nursing team involved. Similarly, when a person is undergoing a serious operation or medical procedure, healing is directed to that person and the whole of the medical team. This may also include other helpers and carers. Cleaners and orderlies too are a vital part of the healing picture.

All such situations greatly benefit from the healing energies summoned up and channelled through the different forms of group work outlined above. In this way Distant Healing very often plays a part in the sacred occasions of birth, death and therapeutic procedure.

Extending your experience

By practising the exercises and carefully evaluating each one, you now have a range of practical ways to develop your experience and confidence. You are equipped to work alone or with a group. So far we have concentrated on working with human subjects, although I have hinted that this could just be the beginning of what you want to do with Distant Healing.

The focus for us, all the way through, has been on the heart centre, the centre that processes all issues of love. But it is first and foremost the place of the Higher Self and the place from which love emanates while you are working as a Distant Healer. I will be returning to emphasise the heart centre's pre-eminence in the final chapter.

I mentioned earlier that Distant Healing works because of Oneness. We are one with every human, every animal, every plant, the whole natural world, the planet and, yes, the rest of the cosmos. Love is Oneness in action. This means that we can extend our work into any of these areas. It also means that, as Distant Healers, we have to consider the activities of humans in relation to themselves and to the rest of the world.

From now on, we have to decide how we are going to respond to violence, crisis and disaster – local, national and global. This is one of the two fundamental issues for all healers in this new century, so I give this special prominence by making it the issue of the penultimate chapter. Before that, let's return to another important and interesting way to extend the work by looking at the whole realm of how to send Distant Healing to animals, plants and the environment. The other fundamental issue of our time concerns this realm.

Part Three

Chapter 11

Working with the environment

We are all connected: each with each, all with all. Not mysticism: just biology.

Moral: as we seek to save the world, so we get closer to saving ourselves.

SIMON BARNES, 'No Island Is An Island' in *Birds* (the magazine of the RSPB), Winter 2006.

The environment calls for our help

As we engage with life, we not only come into energetic contact with other human beings, we also make contact with the mineral, plant and animal worlds. Most of the time we are not aware of these contacts, our consciousness is otherwise engaged. But this is changing; more and more people are recognising our interrelationship with the natural world, how we affect it, and now, more dramatically, how it can affect us. Today, the elemental group energies, of earth, air, fire and water, which shape our environment, are calling out for help.

All life is conscious

We may be used to the presence of an ocean, a river, a lake, a mountain, a hill, a plain, a garden and so on. They are either part of our local landscape or we spend periods of leisure with them. We also make contact with other elemental bodies such as wind, clouds, the warmth and light of the sun, rain, snow and ice. But it is when elemental group energies impact on us that we become much more conscious of them – a stormy sea, a flooding river, a landslide, a hurricane, a forest fire, a volcanic eruption.

The wisdom of indigenous peoples, especially the shamanic, has always acknowledged these forms of consciousness, recognising them as 'beings' in their own right whose collective consciousness is a force or power. This wisdom has come from direct experience of these energetic forms.

But we do not have to belong to a shamanic or indigenous community to commune with natural consciousness. As the celebrated pioneer of interspecies communication, Dorothy Maclean, has shown, it is available to all those who are prepared to open their minds and hearts, enabling the intuitive brow centre. This ability has always been there, but we have denied the subtle sensitivity within us for so long that it has almost become extinct.

During her ground-breaking work as co-founder of the Findhorn Community in Scotland, Dorothy Maclean communicated with the overlighting spiritual forces of plants, the elements and the landscape. These often take the form of group souls or spirits. From these sources, she received numerous beautiful and enlightening transmissions, which became, in effect, dialogues (see, for example, *To Honor the Earth* in Further Reading, page 197). The transmissions indicate that the whole of Nature sees human beings as part of the one web of life in which each part has a unique and vital role. They also demonstrate that, *because all aspects of Creation are conscious, we can communicate with them*. This is a law of energy that has made possible the seemingly wondrous happenings created by healers, holy people and shamanic practitioners throughout the ages.

We hear of the continual extinction of thousands of plant and animal beings, even of certain human groups. With extinction, their energy patterns, and their wisdom, are lost to us. The total effect on our group consciousness is extremely negative. The picture that we currently see is of unhealthy, unbalanced human beings attempting to live in an environment which they are progressively making unhealthy and unbalanced. To restore its state of balance, the environment is 'fighting back', as we are finding to our cost. At a soul level we know what is happening, and the Higher Self is trying to get this awareness through to us. So we are living in a time when there is tremendous pressure from this level to wake up and become aware of the reality of what is happening and to stop living in virtual reality.

Distant Healing, through its understanding of conscious energy, has much to offer in facilitating the changes as species evolve, in preserving those patterns of consciousness in danger of disappearing, and in recovering the wisdom of those that have already disappeared. This is just one form of healing, through which we can offer a vital contribution to the goal of restoring planetary balance and harmony.

Distant Healing is communication with consciousness

The beings that dwell here with us are spiritually and energetically our brothers and sisters. Their energy patterns can be seen by inner vision as patterns of light, like the human pattern of light I described in Chapter 3. The energy pattern that you are merges with the energy pattern of anyone or anything near you. They merge with the light of the ground you both stand on. Your light merges with the light of the air that you breathe and are surrounded by. Your light merges with the energy of the water you drink and with the energy of the food you eat. The whole flow of life is a vast movement of energy and an intricate pattern of light.

The Source, the Light and consciousness are one, and consciousness is what we communicate with. This is why Distant Healers dedicate their work to the Light, work as channels for the Light, put their subjects in the Light, or send Light to those beings and situations that need help. So when Distant Healers utilise the Light through this conscious intention, they are effectively proclaiming: 'Let there be Light!'

Shedding light on the environmental crisis

Many indigenous groups, such as the Native American and the Q'ero people of the Andes, have been speaking about the raising of human consciousness for some three or more decades. By this they mean that there is growing pressure from the spiritual levels for us to acknowledge the spiritual reality of all that is. A natural development of this raising of consciousness is the understanding and acceptance of Oneness.

This may seem new to many, especially to those brought up in certain religions, but the concept of Sacred Unity was always part of many traditions, and it has been the teaching of mystics the world over, not as an intellectual or philosophical notion, but as an existential experience. These traditions may smile at the irony of the 'rediscovery' of Oneness (see, for example, any of the excellent *Conversations With God* series in Further Reading, page 197), but it is still an occasion for celebration and a hope that it has happened in time to begin the unification of human beings with each other and with the natural world.

In the past, the relationship of city-based cultures with Nature was greatly influenced by the doctrine of patriarchal religions and later by the mechanistic world view of rational science. This relationship was based on the premise that human beings were obviously the dominant species with a God-given or inherent right to dominate, subdue and exploit the natural world for human benefit alone. For centuries, this premise was extended by the various colonial powers to indigenous humans: they had to be overcome, subdued and exploited. The same attitude was perpetuated by the Industrial Revolution and its modern offspring of continuous production and technological development – at all costs.

In contrast, early sacred traditions held respect for Nature and its life forms. Human beings were part of an interdependent family of beings in which the natural world was to be co-operated with, not overcome. This co-operation was greatly facilitated by communicating with Nature. As the developed world now faces the global environmental crisis that has arisen through *non-co-operation* with Nature, the raising of consciousness has led to an encouraging determination to engage with the issues.

A range of environmental organisations around the world are working hard to heighten awareness and suggest practical solutions. Universities, colleges and schools are offering degrees and courses in environmental subjects. At the level of the individual, we can now recycle materials, take measures to avoid pollution, try to source our food as locally as possible, become aware of how our own lifestyle impacts on the totality of global effects and make appropriate choices for change. This 'green', eco-friendly agenda implies a new respect for Nature and a movement towards honouring the indigenous wisdom that is still available to us all.

The green agenda for Distant Healing

In most parts of the world, when humans need to relax and de-stress they gravitate towards the green of Nature. When the planet is in balance, plant life returns to its natural place – even when this is a desert. It is no coincidence that the colour of balance is green. When our subtle energy system is in balance, the heart centre vibrates to the colour green. The new agenda for Distant Healing is literally a green one in the sense that it mobilises the soul force of the heart centre to aid the worldwide effort to redress the imbalance that centuries of environmental abuse have brought about.

Again, shamanic cultures have had cause to smile over the scientific debate about whether planet Earth is a living being or not. In the 1960s, scientist James Lovelock proposed the ecological theory that the living matter of the planet functions like a single organism. This was virtually ignored in scientific circles until Lovelock popularised his theory in his books *The Quest for Gaia* (1975), and *Gaia: A New Look at Life on Earth* (1979). Lovelock called this self-regulating system after the Greek goddess Gaia (Earth). Then, after ten years of scientific criticism, Lovelock declared that there was no conscious purpose behind planetary self-regulation. Professor Lynn Margulis, who was principal collaborator with James Lovelock for 25 years, has stressed that Gaia is not an organism or a being (*The Symbiotic Planet: A New Look at Evolution*, 1998). However, New Age, as well as environmental, circles have welcomed the personification of Gaia, seeing it as an assenting, if grudging, nod to indigenous concepts of Earth as mother and nurturer, and certainly a 'being'.

Whatever the debate, transmissions from the natural world, such as those via Dorothy Maclean, indicate that both plant and environmental forces are doing their best to redress the imbalance caused by our activities, even sending healing to us; but they stress that a change to an eco-friendly lifestyle, and sending out healing to the world is what is most needed. This coincides with the entreaties of shamanic populations worldwide to heed the voice of Nature and begin the process of healing without delay. This is also the green heart agenda of Distant Healing.

Communicating with the elements

To work as a Distant Healer with the Earth and the Earth family, you first need to make sure that you can open your lines of communication with them. Our subtle energy system mirrors that of the planet and our need for the right relationship with it begins here. On the physical level, we are composed of all the four essential elements of life, just like the planet. The body is linked to the element earth and the base centre. The various fluids of the body (most of us are composed of around 75 per cent water!) are linked to the element water and the sacral centre. The energy of the animating life force, and the heat of the body, is linked to the element fire and the solar plexus centre. Our breath is linked to the element air, the life force and the heart centre.

It is well known that the ancient esoteric science of astrology also highlights our individual link with the four elements, so that you are an earth, water, fire or air 'sign'. If you are not sure what your element is, look up your sun sign. This comes about through our soul choice of when to be born, which gives each of us an affinity with the relevant element. When you come to working with the environment, make a note of the type of situations or subjects you feel drawn to. Do they tend to be mainly earth-based, or a source of water and so on?

Our physical makeup does mean that what happens to the planet, energetically, is reflected in us, and what happens to us is mirrored in the state of the planet. This is what you will find out when you open your lines of communication to engage with your environment. Communication with the environment begins by acknowledging your relationship with the four elements that go to make it. Let's take this exciting opportunity.

EXERCISE 34

Communing with the Earth

Before Native Americans enter the purification (sweat) lodge, they first give thanks to the Earth in the standing position. Then, in the kneeling position, they honour the Earth by touching the ground with the forehead. This exercise makes use of that formula. If you are unable to take up the bodily positions described, the exercise may still be done through your mental intention and visualisation.

- Stand on the ground with your bare feet a shoulder-width apart, with the knees gently flexed. Use your breathing to relax, but be

exercise continues ▶

totally aware. You are making subtle contact via the energy centres in the soles of the feet. Take six breaths as if you can breathe in the energy of the Earth through the soles of your feet. As you exhale, you share your energies with the Earth.

- Recall an enjoyable walk. Recall the feeling of working with the land. Remember when the sight of a certain landscape gave you joy. All beings come from this Earth and are nourished by it. When you engage with the Earth like this, you are offering your gratitude.

- Now assume a kneeling position, as you honour the Earth. Make a full breath in this position.

- Touch the ground with your forehead (brow centre). This makes contact between the Earth and your visionary self, your intuitive self. Breathe the Earth into your brow centre.

- Now assume a sitting position so that the base of your spine is in contact with the ground. Breathe into the Earth via your base centre.

- From the sitting position, lie down with your back touching the ground. Breathe in the energies of the Earth through the whole of your back. Exhale from your back into the ground.

- Stand up again and relax. When you engage with the Earth like this, you are acknowledging it, and communing with it. See if you can engage in this wordless dialogue.

- As you stand on the ground once again, you appreciate that all visions, all subtle sensations, are grounded in the physical body. This is where you are. The place where you stand is holy ground.

You will have picked up a range of sensations during this exercise. Perhaps Earth spoke to you. As you practise, the range will increase. Make a note of them in your Distant Healing journal. Practise in various locations and note any differences. Now engage with the other three elements.

EXERCISE 35

Communing with Water

Find a natural source of water, which can be large or small.

- Stand or sit near the water source you have chosen (or which has chosen you!). Use your breathing to relax the body. Note everything that this particular source is conveying to you.

- Become aware of your breathing, as you breathe into the sacral centre. Breathe naturally. Water quenches your thirst, and the thirst of the land and plants. Recall a time when you enjoyed drinking simply fresh water. Remember listening to the soothing sound of rain outside. You are communing with the element of Water.

- Allow Water to 'speak' to you. Feel that you can absorb its communication via your sacral centre. Close the exercise with your thanks.

- When you engage with Water like this, you are acknowledging it and communing with it. See if you can engage in this dialogue, which may be without words.

- Practise this exercise with a different source of water. Notice any differences between say, an ocean and a lake, a river and a tiny stream. Remember that other sources like rain, snow, ice or a waterfall can all be engaged with.

EXERCISE 36

Communing with Fire

This exercise can be done in the same way with a fire outdoors or indoors, while you acknowledge the energy of Fire as the release of the energy of the Sun.

exercise continues ▶

- Stand on the ground with your bare feet a shoulder-width apart, with the knees gently flexed. Use your breathing to relax, but be totally aware. Face the direction of the sun (in the morning this is in the east).

- Close your eyes. Become aware of your breathing as you breathe into your solar plexus centre. Visualise that you are able to breathe the light of the sun into this centre. You need the warmth and vitality of the sun. The skin of your body needs its rays to keep you healthy. Remember the feeling of waking up to a sunny day. Recall happy times in the sun. You are communing with the element of Fire. Let your natural rhythm of breath be a 'thank you' to Fire.

- Allow Fire to speak to you.

- As you engage with Fire, allow any feelings to pass by and move on, without comment or judgement.

- Change your body posture and/or location. Note any changes in your communion with Fire.

EXERCISE 37

Communing with Air

If possible, practice this exercise outdoors.

- Stand on the ground with your bare feet a shoulder-width apart, with the knees gently flexed. Use your breathing to relax, but be totally aware.

- Become aware of your breathing as you breathe into your heart centre. Air carries the animating life force and the oxygen that your body needs. It also carries the waste gases that your body discards.

exercise continues ▶

> It carries the scent of the breeze, the flowers, the trees and the smell of the sea. You are communing with the element of Air. Let your natural rhythm of breath be a 'thank you' to Air. Allow Air to speak to you.
>
> - How does Air move right now? What does this feel like?
> - Change your body position and/or location. Note any changes in your communion with Air.

From a Distant Healing point of view, the great need for environmental healing stems from the disruption of energetic flow and the millions of disconnections in the energy web that links it with us humans and the rest of the Earth family. This is what you need to be aware of when you feel motivated to work with the environment. One of the single most devastating causes of the disruption of energy flow is the sense of separation from the natural world that humans feel. This has resulted in the breakdown of relationship.

The list of disconnections is long and you could create your own. They allow us to do things to the environment, such as gouge a way through the land for a new road, in such a way that the energy flow of the land, and all the beings dwelling on it, is interrupted. A simple ceremony of thanking and honouring would have gone a long way to repairing the energy web. This is where Distant Healing has much to offer.

The exercises above not only help you to acknowledge your link with the four elements of the environment, they also help you to reconnect with them. Now you need to look at how they compose the natural world around you. Become aware of the climate, the movement of air and water, the ground beneath your feet, the features of the landscape and the signs of the seasons. Even if you live in the middle of a city, it is rooted in Nature and depends on it. You breathe the air of the city, you drink the water, your food was grown somewhere. You need sources of warmth to stay alive. Now it is time to engage with your landscape.

EXERCISE 38
Engaging with your landscape

- Go somewhere outdoors where you can sit comfortably. Take a few full breaths to help you relax your body. The object of the exercise is to be fully relaxed, while at the same time being fully aware.

- Now attune to what is before you, beginning with the light. Become aware of what is nearby. What can you see?

- Close your eyes and listen. What do you hear?

- Pay attention to stillness, birdsong, rustlings and movement, to the feel of the air and the feeling of the day, the behaviour of the clouds and so on.

- As you honour each part of the life around you, you expand your boundaries on all levels. This deepens your perception of, and alignment with, healing energies.

- Regular practice of this exercise will reveal many life secrets.

The disrupted landscape and oceans

If you took a trip to a landscape that is special to you, you probably noticed places that had been disrupted in some way: a new road, a housing development, a factory project, etc. All such operations involve energetic disruption. Furthermore, they usually involve a range of polluting factors. Aboriginal people would tell you that none of these things were done 'in a sacred manner', by acknowledging our oneness with the land. Instead the attitude is that the land is there to be used; it has no consciousness or feelings.

Yet, if you brought one of those sights to mind and held your hands up to see if healing was needed, your hands would probably signal that it was. Recall how I started Distant Healing with the Italian granddad. My inner urge was to help and my hands knew what to do. If the old man had not needed help, my hands would not have responded.

The next exercise deals with how you can respond to an environmental challenge, whether this is a local need or a global problem. Near where I live a new highway is being built. When this two-year project is completed, it is hoped that the traffic on this busy route will flow more quickly and freely. The work has meant digging out huge swathes of land that have to be dumped somewhere else. Trees have been cut down and natural habitats destroyed.

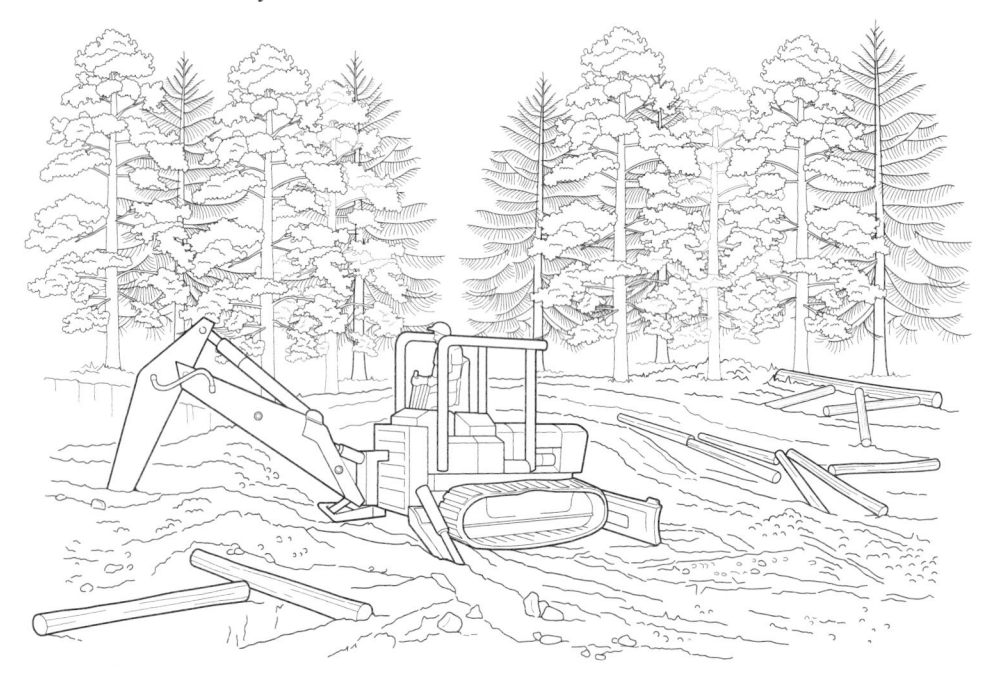

Figure 23. A disrupted landscape

No one, like an indigenous person might do, 'asks' the land how it feels about this, apologises for the damage, or makes an offering in recompense. A great deal of energetic turmoil has been released which will have to be balanced in some way. This is where Distant Healing comes in.

You may feel more inspired to help with some environmental problem you have seen on TV or in the newspapers, which is farther away from home. This is just as important. I emphasise, all through this book, to go with what you are drawn to; this is what you are equipped to deal with; this is your personal challenge.

Perhaps you feel drawn to work with environmental issues. Your help is certainly needed. Simply attune as usual and set to work in the way you have been practising so far. By applying the method in the next exercise, you will soon find that you have arrived at a special way of working with the bigger global problems.

EXERCISE 39
Responding to an environmental issue – sending out healing Light

- Either work on one situation (which has preferably chosen you) or more if you feel inclined. You may need to make a list, just as you did for other subjects. Make sure the phone is disconnected and that you will not be disturbed. Attune your work space and attune yourself as you have already practised.

- You may wish to light a candle as a symbol of the Light of the Source. If so, dedicate it to the work and to any helpers you might have in the spiritual realms. Give thanks that you have been given the opportunity to send out healing Light to the environment.

- Bring your focus to your heart centre. As you inhale, visualise this centre filling with the Light. With the next breath, the Light fills your chest.

- Allow the particular environmental issue to be brought to mind. You may be surprised by the aspect that is presented to you. Avoid judgement. Ask for the Light to be sent out to the issue you mention. You can say aloud or in your mind: 'I ask for healing to be sent to (the presenting issue).'

- If you have a list of issues, ask for the Light to be sent out to each subject as you mention them one by one. Carefully work through your list like this. Take your time. If you feel the need to pause, do so. This simply means that you are in tune with what is happening energetically.

- When you reach the end of your list, give thanks.

exercise continues ▶

- Rest assured that the particular issue, or issues, have received healing that is most needed at this time. Sit quietly with your experience.

- When you have completed your work, blow out the candle. This can be done by sending out the light of the candle. Pause for a moment and see if you intuitively feel where it needs to go. This is usually the first place that comes to mind. As you blow out the candle, say: 'I send the Light out to –.'

- Once you have closed your session, you have handed over the work to higher powers. It is time to stop thinking about it.

In the early stages of practice, alternate the first basic technique of sending out the Light (as above) with the second basic technique of creating the Light pool or circle. This follows next.

EXERCISE 40

Responding to an environmental issue – creating the Light pool

- Either work on one situation (which has preferably chosen you) or more if you feel inclined. You may need to make a list, just as you did for other subjects. Make sure the phone is disconnected and that you will not be disturbed. Attune your work space and attune yourself as you have already practised.

- You may wish to light a candle as a symbol of the Light of healing. If so, dedicate it to the work and to any helpers you might have in the spiritual realms. Give thanks that you have been given the opportunity to help the environment through the Light of Distant Healing.

exercise continues ▶

- Bring your focus to your heart centre. As you inhale, visualise this centre filling with Light. With the next breath, the Light fills your chest.

- Now see this Light extending from you to a place in front of you to make an energy pool or circle.

- As you bring your chosen issue to mind, ask for it to be put in the Light. You can say aloud or in your mind: 'I ask for healing for (name the issue).' If you have a list of issues, ask for them to be put in the Light, mentioning them one by one. Carefully work through your list like this. Take your time. If you feel the need to pause, do so. This simply means that you are in tune with what is happening energetically.

- Visualise that the issue, or issues, have been gathered into the Light pool or circle. Here, they will receive the healing they need most at this time. Sit quietly with your experience.

- When you have completed your work, give thanks and blow out the candle. This can be done by sending out the light of the candle. Pause for a moment and see if you intuitively feel where it needs to go. This is usually the first place that comes to mind. As you blow out the candle, say: 'I send the Light out to –.'

- Once you have closed your session, you have handed over the work to higher powers. It is time to stop thinking about it.

As before, if you wish to follow a session like those above with some other spiritual practice, you are in the ideal state to do this. If not, realise that the work has opened your energy centres more than is needed for everyday functioning. In other words, you no longer need to be open to that level of energy flow. Carry out the essential Closing-down Procedure that you have already learned in Chapter 5, on pages 56–7.

Some Distant Healers are so sensitive that they absorb incompatible energies from the environmental situations that they have been working with. Here, the clearing exercise in the Closing-down Procedure is called for. When your Distant Healing session is in the evening, the Closing-down Procedure also ensures sound sleep. Remember that 'closing down' refers to a procedure that returns your subtle energy system to everyday functioning; it is linked to your closing your working sessions. It does not mean fully closing the energy centres or shutting down any of the body systems.

Carrying out the Closing-down Procedure after each session of work will eventually become second nature. You can also use it to return your subtle energy system to everyday functioning at other times too. Even a conversation or reading a book about spiritual or environmental matters can open your centres. And this is what can happen when you work with a group.

Environmental work with a group

Group work can be carried out in exactly the same way as set out in Chapter 6 for the Distant Healing Circle (Exercises 19 and 20, pages 62 and 64). You may even find that the group mixes in environmental issues with other subjects. It is up to the group as a whole to choose how to work. Sometimes a special session devoted exclusively to the environment is a powerful way to highlight the issues in everybody's mind. The energies of the solstices and equinoxes are especially conducive to this form of healing work. Once the programme for a session is agreed, stick to it so that everyone knows what they will be doing.

Chapter **12**

Working with plants and animals

Plants as teachers and healers

This is a teaching book but, as you follow it, your experience becomes your own teaching. Teaching comes from within and without. Once you have spent time with the environment, it won't be long before it sends out a challenge to your inner teacher: are you listening to your inner voice? As sages down the centuries have acknowledged, Nature, too, is our teacher.

The fossil record shows that plants were the first to begin colonising the planet and that this process began in the sea. As we look at the plant world today, we could easily forget their underwater beginnings, but these have ensured their intimate relationship with water. Plants have since formed the nutritional basis for the life of insects and all other animals, including ourselves. Most plants have the ability to combine the energy of the sun with air, water and minerals from the Earth to create their stems, leaves, flowers, pollen, fruits, nuts, tubers, roots – which animals, including humans, consume. The plant realm has also provided the basis for the development of the pharmaceutical products used in medicine and health care today. But communication with the plants could reveal even more of their healing abilities and intimate structures without our having to dissect them.

Most people's connection with plants is with a garden or window box, or by taking a walk in the park. But in past times we were intimately involved with them, especially during food production. For example, the journey of a loaf of bread to the table began with the sower going out to sow the seed. Then groups of agricultural workers joined in the harvesting by hand, stacking the sheaves of straw and winnowing the grain. This was taken to the mill to be ground into flour and put in sacks. Flour was made available for households or bakers to buy, and the housewife or the baker would make the loaves by hand and bake them. In the developed world, each of these steps in the production of bread has been mechanised, so that many children think that bread is simply something sliced in a packet that you buy in a supermarket. They are totally unaware of how it got there. Where people eat other staple plant foods, there is a similar trend towards mechanisation, with a loss of connection with the growing and production process.

The mechanisation of food production is undoubtedly in many ways a human benefit, but the intervention of machines affects the food energetically. To test this, hold a pendulum over any food that you have bought and it will show a negative swing. Or hold your hands over it and you will feel them sending out energy, often healing energy, to the food product. This means that all those activities where plants come into contact with machines would benefit from Distant Healing. If we use the road-building scenario, Distant Healing is also needed where plants have been uprooted or destroyed, and the energy flow interrupted. Very often you will find that when something destructive happens to plants, the group energy needs healing on behalf of the individuals.

I have a friend who feels pain whenever she sees a truck loaded with felled trees. She senses the effects of the felling and trimming that has not been done 'in a sacred manner'. She feels compelled to send healing to the trees already cut up for transport to the sawmill, as well as the ground where they were once growing, and the other trees left behind.

Your Distant Healing work will always be needed for individual plants, gardens, plantations and any locations where it is necessary to repair the damage caused by local projects. But, as with the mineral environment, there are now global issues that concern the plant realm. The destruction of the world's rain forests, for example, is already having various catastrophic effects. These vast ecosystems act as the lungs of the planet, giving out oxygen and taking in carbon dioxide. They also absorb the rain that now falls in a destructive way on barren earth.

The overlighting spirits of plant groups have much help to offer us humans, but, having failed to communicate with them, we are missing these opportunities. However, all is not lost. Distant Healing, which honours and celebrates the plants, will take us all a step forward towards a new and more positive relationship with them. The next two exercises will help you to do just that.

> **EXERCISE 41**
>
> *Engaging with the plant world*
>
> You can of course commune with plants in pots, even bunches of flowers in a store, but, if possible, go to a place outdoors where there are plants.
>
> - Sit comfortably. Use your breathing to relax the body. Breathe naturally.
>
> - Allow your gaze to relax as you look towards the plants around you. Wait patiently until you feel that a plant or plants are calling to you in some way.
>
> - Still relaxed, pay attention to this plant or group of plants. Allow them to 'speak' to you. Keep an open mind and suspend your tendency to judgement. Try to simply listen with your full attention.
>
> - When you sense that the communication is over, thank the plants and allow some time to sit with your experience.
>
> - Make a note in your journal. Try the exercise in other locations.

Now we will communicate with a single tree. Trees provide beautiful examples of beings with their heads in the heavens and their roots deep in the soil of the Earth – a lesson in grounding the spiritual in the physical. Some trees are many hundreds of years old and have the 'wisdom' that comes with their great age.

EXERCISE 42

Listening to a tree

Go to a place outdoors where there are trees. They can be any size. Older trees have much to communicate about life on this planet.

- Stand or sit in the landscape and wait for a tree to 'call' to you, or focus on one that you feel attracted to. This will happen if you are patient. Either sit close to this tree or stand with your back against it.

- Use your breathing to relax. Wait for the tree to communicate with you.

- Keep an open mind and suspend your tendency to judgement. Try to simply listen with your full attention.

- When you sense that the communication is over, thank the tree and allow some time to sit with your experience.

- Make a note in your journal. Try the exercise with other trees.

This can be a very productive exercise to do with a group, where members can hold hands around the tree. Later, individual experiences can be shared and group learning enhanced. The same applies to the next exercise.

EXERCISE 43

Sending Distant Healing to the plant world

Follow the techniques you have already learned if you wish to work solo. Here is an example of an advanced technique where you find yourself working with the plants in a large garden. In such a case, it is important not to decide beforehand what needs your help, but to

exercise continues ▶

go with the flow of the healing. The working scenario would be similar if you were 'taken to', say, a large forest.

Though you always work with the subject, rather than the condition, in astral level work you will often be aware of your hands moving into the area of a stated condition, as well as other important sites. Go with the flow of your guidance and make a note of what happens later. Note: this exercise is formatted for indoor practice but could just as easily be conducted outside.

- Prepare and dedicate your working space. Make sure that you will not be interrupted in any way. Have your subject, or list of subjects to hand. Attune, light your candle and dedicate the work. Ask to be used as a channel for healing, and to be guided by your Higher Self (soul). You will look forward to being directed by this source (whether or not you will be doing any Distant Healing at the astral level).

- Sit with your feet flat on the floor or ground with your hands, palms up, on your thighs or in your lap. The hands should not overlap or touch. (In astral work it is essential for the palm centres to remain active, hence the palms-up position of the hands.) Use the breath to calm and relax the body. Let go of any worries or anxieties with the out-breath, through the open mouth. When you feel attuned, close your mouth and breathe normally. Check that your body is relaxed, including the back of the neck, the shoulders and pelvis. Sit in the silence for a few moments.

- Now put the garden in your mind's eye. Mention it by name because the vibration of the name strengthens your link (as in the Healing Triangle).

- Close your eyes to aid concentration and wait quietly and patiently to see if you become aware that a place in the garden is in front of you. If you have been 'taken' to the garden, you will sense this. It becomes easier when you relax and accept that it is possible for this to happen.

exercise continues ▶

- Allow your intuitive guidance to help you sense where your hands need to go.

- If this is what the plant needs, you will feel healing energy leave your hands, or whatever sign tells you that you are working. Keep them over the area until you feel a change in the flow of energy, which could be sensed as a marked decrease, or falling off, in intensity. The signal is that all, or part, of the healing is complete.

- Wait for your guidance to see if you need to give healing elsewhere. There may be another plant or plants that you need to work with.

- The energetic activity in your hands is confirmation that this is not taking place in your imagination. A person with developed perceptions would be able to sense or 'see' what was going on and confirm that you were working this way.

- As you complete your work with each plant, mentally thank it. Now take a full breath and, as you exhale, surround it with a protective sphere of light. This may be done mentally or by raising your arms and moving your hands gently to make a sphere around the astral body in front of you.

- When you sense that your work in the garden is complete, relax and allow yourself to return to your physical body.

- Send out the light of the candle. Pause for a moment and see if you intuitively feel where it needs to go. This is usually the first place that comes to mind. As you blow out the candle, say: 'I send the Light out to –.'

- Carry out the Closing-down Procedure outlined in Chapter 5, pages 56–7.

Group work with plants

The needs of the plant realm are an ideal subject for group work. Create your sessions in the usual way. Again, it makes the routine more interesting to have a special session devoted to plants and trees. Similarly, members may come to the meeting one day with particular concerns that they would like the group to address.

Working with the animal realm

Animals and plants are constantly caught up in many forms of environmental pollution and devastation: oil and chemical discharge, and numerous forms of waste disposal, into the sea, rivers and on land, for example. They also suffer from the destruction and pollution caused by human conflict. Everything that has been said about the environment and plants also applies to the animals. They too experience interruptions to their energy flow, especially on a group basis. Animals are as susceptible to disease and injury as a result of energetic interruption as all other living beings. Many wild animals are under threat of extinction as their habitats become increasingly unviable.

Millions of animals and birds are eaten every year without a sense of gratitude from their human consumers. I recently saw a travel documentary about an idyllic island. The tourists loved to go to the market to buy souvenirs and soak up the atmosphere. In one place you could buy the freshest chicken, alive in their wooden cages. Seated next to them was a man with a wooden block and a chopper. Once you had ordered your chicken, he would reach into the cage, put the chicken's head on the block and chop it off in front of the other chickens!

Back home you can see a truck filled to bursting with animals bound for the abattoir. There they will queue up to be slaughtered and this will not be done 'in a sacred manner', with gratitude. Distant Healing is needed in all such situations. Blessing and thanking your food can also become a vital Distant Healing activity.

Animals as teachers and healers

On a summer's day in 1995, I found the dead body of a green woodpecker on the doorstep of our house. Marvelling at its beautiful plumage and sorry about its demise, I buried it in the vegetable garden. Later that night, the spirit of the woodpecker communicated with me for over a half-hour. Woodpecker said that all things had the capacity to teach. As if my chest were the trunk of a tree, Woodpecker bored into it. 'You see, I will bore a way through your chest to let the light in and the energy of your heart out!' Was there a link with the green colour of its feathers? I wondered. Woodpecker told how it communes with the trees and understands them.

This knowledge is available to all, through communication with Woodpecker. Towards the end of our 'conversation', Woodpecker described the meaning of fame: 'When you are looked up to, your job is to reflect back the Great Spirit. This is the only purpose of being looked up to, so that *you* send back the image of spiritual truth.'

Two years later, I received an intriguing message from a particular magpie that lives with its family in a pine near my home. This was about how the message of love was carried by the birds in colour and sound. Even a lowly fly once told me some dazzling stories about multiple sight. The wonder of all the communications I have received from the animal realm is that they seem totally relevant to everyone's life, yet they were couched in a way that also had personal significance for me. This is why I encourage you to commune with the animals. But also because it will greatly enhance your work with them as a Distant Healer. Many owners tell of conversations with their pets and how their pets often seem to know their innermost thoughts. So, although you may have an animal you are fond of, the next exercise needs to be with an animal you have never met.

EXERCISE 44

Communing with the animal realm

- Go somewhere outdoors where you can sit comfortably. Take a few full breaths to help you relax your body. The object of the exercise is to be fully relaxed, while at the same time being fully aware.

- Now attune to what is before you. This means putting your mind in the heart centre while you allow your relaxed gaze to look into the distance. Also become aware of what is nearby.

exercise continues ▶

- Pay attention to stillness, birdsong, rustlings and movement, to the feel of the air and the feeling of the day, and so on.
- If you live in an urban setting, you can train yourself to hear beyond the sounds of traffic, etc.
- Close your eyes and listen. What do you hear?
- Allow yourself to 'hear' the voice of an animal or bird in your environment. Be patient, in active waiting mode (the opposite of just passing the time).
- This is a way of honouring the animal life around you. It deepens your perception of, and alignment with the animals, on all levels. Before leaving, give your thanks.
- Regular practice of this exercise will reveal many life secrets.
- Make a note of your experience in your journal. You can decide whether it is appropriate for you to share it with other people or your Distant Healing group. When you can, sharing is always a way of learning.

Domestic animals and pets

Like all life forms, animals respond to love and lovelessness. All animals are sensitive to their owner's state of health and well-being because they are able to pick this up on all levels. As with human situations, there are a number of occasions when Distant Healing is appropriate and ideal for animal subjects. Some may be too dangerous to approach, either because they are wild, or their injury prevents contact, or they are inaccessible.

You may get requests to send healing to domestic animals and pets in the same way as you would for human subjects. In some countries, the treatment of animals is the sole preserve of veterinary surgeons. So, for example, hands-on healing is only practised with the full permission of the vet. There are, however, no such restrictions for Distant Healers. Send your healing help just as you did in the baseline exercises of Chapter 5, pages 53–7.

When you receive a request to send healing to a sick animal, you may find that you are called upon to wait and see if you are going to work on the astral level. If so, your work may proceed along the lines of the following.

EXERCISE 45
Working with a sick animal – astral level healing

Animals are very open and receptive to this form of healing. Though you always work with the subject, rather than the condition, in astral level work you will often be aware of your hands moving into the area of a stated condition, as well as other important sites such as the centres. Go with the flow of your guidance and make a note of what happens later.

- Make sure that you will not be interrupted in any way. Prepare and dedicate your working space. Have your list of subjects to hand. Attune, light your candle and dedicate the work. Ask to be used as a channel for healing, and to be guided by your Higher Self (soul). You will look forward to being directed by this source (whether or not you will be doing any Distant Healing at the astral level).

- Sit with your feet flat on the floor with your hands, palms up, on your thighs or in your lap. The hands should not overlap or touch. (In astral work it is essential for the palm centres to remain active, hence the palms-up position of the hands.)

- Use the breath to calm and relax the body. Let go of any worries or anxieties with the out-breath, through the open mouth. When you feel attuned, close your mouth and breathe normally. Check that your body is relaxed, including the back of the neck, the shoulders and pelvis. Sit in the silence for a few moments.

- Now focus on the request for help. Mention the subject by name (if it has one) because the vibration of the name strengthens your link with the animal (as in the Healing Triangle, see page 12).

exercise continues ▶

- Close your eyes to aid concentration and wait quietly and patiently to see if you become aware that the subject is in front of you.

- If you have been 'taken' to the animal, or it has been 'brought' to you, you will sense this. This becomes easier when you relax and accept that it is possible for this to happen. You will also be able to sense whether the animal is lying or sitting in front of you and how the body is orientated.

- Mentally make sure that you are comfortably orientated to carry out what needs to be done. Allow your intuitive guidance to help you sense where your hands need to go.

- Let's take an example as illustration. Your help has been requested for a cat which has become ill. In this case, once you are aware of the cat's astral body in front of you, you will probably feel drawn to put your hands over the area in question. If this is what it needs, you will feel healing energy leave your hands, or whatever sign tells you that you are working. Keep them over the area until you feel a change in the flow of energy, which could be sensed as a marked decrease, or falling off, in intensity. The signal is that all, or part, of the healing is complete.

- Wait for your guidance to see if you need to give healing elsewhere. There may be a centre involved, for example, or you may need to move your hands to somewhere else.

- The energetic activity in your hands is confirmation that this is not taking place in your imagination. A person with developed perceptions would be able to sense or 'see' what was going on and confirm that you were working this way.

- When you have completed your work, mentally thank the cat. Now take a full breath and, as you exhale, surround it with a protective sphere of light. This may be done mentally or by raising your arms and moving your hands gently to make a sphere around the astral body in front of you (as in Figure 21, page 120).

exercise continues ▶

- At this point, either the cat returns to its physical body, or you return to your physical body.

- (Where there is another subject to work with, you may also remain in the astral body state to receive the next subject on your list in the same way.)

- If there is another subject to work with, first make sure that the one you were working on is no longer in front of you (it has returned to its physical body). Now visualise clearing silver light washing over your upraised palms. You can now proceed to the next subject on your list. Take a short pause if you feel the need.

- Follow the same procedure as before. Finally break your link with the last subject by clearing your hands.

- When you have completed your work, blow out the candle. This can be done by sending out the light of the candle. Pause for a moment and see if you intuitively feel where it needs to go. This is usually the first place that comes to mind. As you blow out the candle, say: 'I send the Light out to –.'

- Carry out the Closing-down Procedure outlined in Chapter 5.

The death of an animal

A common situation where Distant Healing is called for occurs when a pet animal is dying or passing over. Sadness and a sense of loss surrounds the passing of a pet, but in terms of a life journey, the animal, just like a human person, is dropping off the body and continuing life without it – the life that was there before the body.

Here, the Distant Healer is joining the animal on this part of their journey, so the request for help over a passing, or terminal, illness is an honour. It also helps the veterinary team that has the job of putting the animal down. Lastly, it should be sent to the owner who is going to suffer distress at the death of the animal. This is the subject of the next exercise.

If you find that you are affected by cases like these, you will find help by looking at Chapter 9, pages 99–112, again.

EXERCISE 46

Sending healing to a dying animal

In this scenario, you have been told that a friend's dog is very sick and cannot benefit from further treatment. In order to end its suffering, it is going to be put down. The friend asks you to send healing.

- Make sure the phone is disconnected and that you will not be disturbed. Attune both your work space and yourself.

- You may wish to light a candle as a symbol of the Light of healing. If so, dedicate it to the work and any helpers you might have in the spiritual realms. Give thanks that you have been given the opportunity to send out healing Light.

- Bring your focus to your heart centre. As you inhale, visualise this centre filling with the Light. With the next breath, the Light fills your chest.

- Ask for the Light to be sent out to the dog. You can say aloud or in your mind: 'I ask for healing to be sent to (name).' Offer your thanks.

- (When you have a list of animal subjects, carefully work through your list like this. Take your time. If you feel the need to pause, do so. This simply means that you are in tune with what is happening energetically. When you reach the end of your list, give thanks.)

- Rest assured that healing Light has been sent to where it is needed. Sit quietly with your experience.

- When you have completed your work, blow out the candle. This can be done by sending out the light of the candle. Pause for a moment and see if you intuitively feel where it needs to go. As you blow out the candle, say: 'I send the Light out to –.'

exercise continues ▶

- Once you have closed your session, you have handed over the list to higher powers. It is time to stop thinking about the case.

Don't forget your Closing-down Procedure, Chapter 5, pages 56–7. You could alternate similar cases with the Light pool technique below. In this case, death is the result of an accident.

EXERCISE 47
Creating the Light pool for a dying animal

In this case, you have been contacted by someone at a racecourse. A horse has had a serious accident and must be put down. Allow your intuition to help you create a list of subjects, beginning with the horse. You might want to include the rider, the owner and all those who witnessed the accident and subsequent injury to the horse.

- Make sure the phone is disconnected and that you will not be disturbed. Attune your work space and yourself as before.

- You may wish to light a candle as a symbol of the Light of healing. If so, dedicate it to the work and any helpers you might have in the spiritual realms. Give thanks that you have been given the opportunity to help others through the Light of Distant Healing.

- Bring your focus to your heart centre. As you inhale, visualise this centre filling with Light. With the next breath, the Light fills your chest.

- Now see this Light extending from you to a place in front of you to make an energy pool or circle.

- As you look over your list, ask for those on it to be put in the Light, mentioning them one by one. You can say this aloud or in your mind: 'I ask for healing for (name).' Carefully work through your

exercise continues ▶

list like this. Take your time, pausing if necessary. This simply means that you are in tune with what is happening energetically.

- When you reach the end of your list, give thanks.
- Visualise that all those on the list have been gathered into the Light pool or circle. Here, they will receive healing they need. Sit quietly with your experience.
- When you have completed your work, blow out the candle. This can be done by sending out the light of the candle. Pause for a moment and see if you intuitively feel where it needs to go. As you blow out the candle, say: 'I send the Light out to –.'

Once you have closed your session, you have handed over the list to higher powers. It is time to stop thinking about the case.

Honouring your work

You will have found that animals, plants and the landscape are gateways to other states of consciousness. Their teaching is that they are co-partners with us in shaping the living environment. Careful study of your journal entries may show how a pattern of work is emerging that demonstrates your unique affinity with certain aspects of the Earth and/or the Earth family. If you work with a Distant Healing group, a way of honouring the work can be for each member to tell their Earth story.

EXERCISE 48

Telling your Earth story

- After your Distant Healing work, break up into groups of three or four.

exercise continues ▶

- When it is your turn, tell the small group about a particular life experience in which you felt the presence of the natural world.

- Some members have felt pain over what is befalling the planet and its natural inhabitants. In the words of the celebrated Vietnamese Zen master, Thich Nhat Hanh, they have 'heard the Earth crying'.

- Listen to each account with compassion and full attention, watching for signs of your own 'tuning out'.

- Let silence surround each Earth story.

- Recreate the circle and pass the Love round to end the session.

To deal with the second of the two crucial issues of our time, we are certainly going to need some unconditional love. But the most empowering thing for us, as Distant Healers, is that we can beam this healing Love into those violent situations, and the family, societal, political and economic issues that are crying out for help in every part of our planet. In the next chapter we will look at how to set about doing this.

Chapter **13**

Taking action to heal local and global issues

The polarisation of human behaviour

As far as the natural world is concerned, the raising of human consciousness cannot happen soon enough. However, as the pressure for change increases, it is tending to polarise people. Some *are* becoming more spiritually aware, and want to implement lifestyle choices accordingly, while the response of others ranges from the apathetic and despairing to the violent and chaotic. We are witnessing this polar reaction now and this is what is creating important new challenges for Distant Healing.

Somewhere in the middle of the two poles of consciousness is a general feeling of separation. This is the destructive expansion of the sense of separation from others and the natural world. People no longer feel part of a family, their friends, their local community, their nation, and few have ever considered themselves as part of the global community.

Many human activities encourage separation, especially those of political, religious, nationalistic and ethnic groups. Nearer to home, we are separated by lifestyle, income, gender, sexuality, age, disability and the way we appear to others. The media constantly report on the impact of these divisions so that they are further imprinted on our minds. Our oneness with each other should mean that we enjoy and celebrate difference. Instead, difference is used to encourage one group to feel superior to another, and to provide the excuse to denigrate and exploit others. Very often these conditioned attitudes are backed by so-called sacred texts or traditional cultural norms, making communication nearly impossible or very difficult.

One of the problems with polarisation is that this becomes the great divide, with each polarity fearing and hating the other, and wanting to further emphasise difference rather than reach out with compassion and understanding.

The energetic problem is even deeper. As with the effects of disruption on the natural world, polarisation and separation among human beings is creating serious interruptions to energy flow. This, in turn, creates a chronic malaise in the global population which manifests as disease, despair, fear and violence. These effects are mirrored in such environmental problems as drought, famine, earthquake, destructive climate change and so on.

The challenge for Distant Healers

Our own sense of helplessness often stems from feelings that the things we hear about are always beyond our control – a war-torn country, extreme cruelty meted out to the innocent, a frightening mechanical disaster, etc. – because they are happening in other parts of the world. But, sooner or later, the repercussions of these happenings will come knocking on our door, and we will ignore them at our peril. Years ago it was happening to *them* and they were far away. But now it is happening in our neighbourhood.

We know all about these things because the media are very good at reporting them. Nevertheless, as Distant Healers, we want to do something. After all, what is the point of helping the people on our healing list if we do nothing to help those bruised and battered societies in which they and others live and are part of our world too? Distant Healing offers everyone in every society the opportunity to become empowered to do both.

The network of consciousness

The unified field theory is believed by quantum mechanics scientists to connect everything in the universe, including gravity, nuclear reactions, electromagnetic forces and human consciousness. Modern physics, then, supports the findings of Distant Healing that thought forms, such as ideas and information, are able to travel from one part of the human family to another, via a network of consciousness (the unified field of science). It explains how negative thoughts and information are having such a disastrous effect on the human psyche, but it is also the clue to positive action. The network of consciousness operates unconditionally and energetic transactions move in all directions. Recall that the network of consciousness facilitates your being able to send healing Light to anywhere in the universe. We can take good advantage of this in planning how to use Distant Healing to heal the effects of fear and hatred.

The plan of action

I suggest that you begin with a twofold plan. First, start with your own locality. Send out healing Light into it, or, send out to specific local needs. Second, keep the big picture in mind by simply observing what is going on, without judgement or thinking about how a certain problem should be solved. This is the same attitude you used earlier on in your Distant Healing practice where I encouraged you to be open to the guidance of your intuitive wisdom, or Higher Self.

Then allow a situation to call to you, just as you did with elements of the landscape, the plants and animals. When you become aware of this call, it is because you are equipped to deal with the situation at that point in time and your healing contribution is needed. The exercises that follow are suggestions for practice and should be modified to suit your own, or your group's, needs.

EXERCISE 49

Sending Light into a locality

First check how you feel about the situation that you want to work with and what you think about it. Use your breathing to calm and relax yourself. Your healing request should be unconditional. Do not decide in advance what you think should happen in this locality. This

exercise continues ▶

allows decisions to be made at the level of the Higher Self. Remember, healing energy, like prayer, travels at the level of the intentional thought.

- Make sure the phone is disconnected and that you will not be disturbed. Attune both your work space and yourself as outlined in previous chapters.

- You may wish to light a candle as a symbol of the Light of the Source. If so, dedicate it to the work and any helpers you might have in the spiritual realms. Give thanks that you have been given the opportunity to send out healing Light.

- Bring your focus to your heart centre. As you inhale, visualise this centre filling with the Light. With the next breath, the Light fills your chest.

- Ask for the Light to be sent out to the locality you specify. You can say aloud or in your mind: 'I ask for healing to be sent to (name).'

- If you are sending out to more than one locality, ask for the Light to be sent out to each locality as you mention them one by one. Carefully work through your list, taking your time and pausing if necessary. This means that you are in tune with what is happening energetically.

- When you reach the end of your list, give thanks. Sit quietly with your experience.

- Rest assured that healing Light has been sent to where it is needed.

- When you have completed your work, blow out the candle. This can be done by sending out the light of the candle. Pause for a moment and see if you intuitively feel where it needs to go. As you blow out the candle, say: 'I send the Light out to –.'

- Once you have closed your session, relax and realise that you have handed over the situation(s) to higher powers.

TAKING ACTION TO HEAL LOCAL AND GLOBAL ISSUES • 169

EXERCISE 50

Sending Light to a disaster situation – the Distant Healing Circle

The group has agreed that if there is a report of a disaster or situation that they would like to address, this is what the focus of the session will be. In this case, the situation was reported on TV that day.

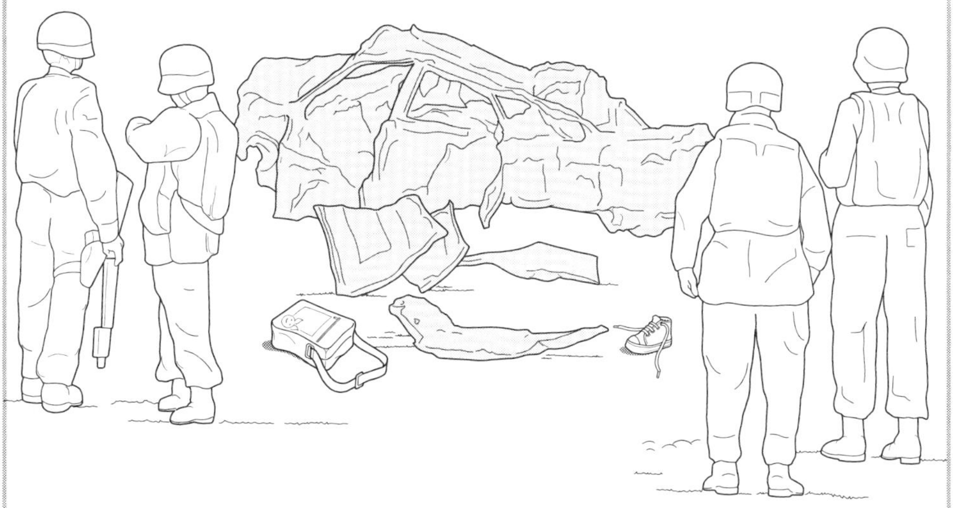

Figure 24. A disaster situation

Disconnect all telephones. Have a circle of chairs in the centre of which is a small table with a candle and some matches. Members might like to add items symbolising healing, and so on. Where possible, the group should sit with male next to female, experienced next to inexperienced. By alternating genders, the energies of the Circle are easier to balance. This also applies to alternating experienced with inexperienced members.

The chosen leader should open the meeting with a welcome and help the group to attune, and then facilitate the Distant Healing.

- The leader's role is to make sure that everyone is in the best possible state to work. It may be necessary, therefore, for the group

exercise continues ▶

to first discuss the report. This helps the group to focus after covering the various aspects of the report in discussion.

- The group sits in a circle with feet flat on the floor, and the hands, palms up, on their thighs, or in their laps without linking. The leader instructs the group as follows:

- 'Take six breaths to calm and relax the body, letting go of any worries or anxieties with the out-breath, through the open mouth. Close the mouth, when you feel attuned, and breathe normally.'

- 'Check that the body is relaxed, including the back of the neck, the shoulders and pelvis. Close your eyes and allow the calm silence to settle.'

- The leader lights the candle and dedicates the light to the work of the Circle, asking for protection and soul guidance. The leader continues:

- 'The light of the candle is the Light of the Source of healing. Breathe it into the heart centre. Allow the Light to fill your chest.'

- 'Now pass the energy in your heart centre to the person on your left so that you are all linked together.' Intuitively, you may have to wait a moment to gather your heart energy before you can pass on.

- The leader should be aware of this and allow enough time for group linking, for this is the foundation of the circle. With practice, it is possible to sense when energetic linking is complete.

- With the Circle ready, the leader expresses the purpose of the meeting and gives thanks, on behalf of the group, for the opportunity to be of service. The group healing request should be unconditional. This allows decisions about outcomes to be made at the level of the Higher Self. Remember, healing energy, like prayer, travels at the level of the intentional thought.

exercise continues ▶

- With this in mind, the leader asks for healing Light to be sent to the situation. A simple form of this could be: 'We ask for healing to be sent to (state the situation without adding opinions or judgement).'

- The group sits together in silence. It is important to realise that the group's intention, motivated by love, has enabled the Light of healing to be sent to the situation.

- The leader gives time for quiet reflection and then indicates that the sending-out process is complete with a verbal signal such as 'Thank you'.

- After a short break, the group can discuss the work of the Circle, share experiences and queries to consolidate learning.

- The work may be followed by another spiritual activity such as meditation, a reading, or listening to music.

- Finally, the leader closes the Healing Circle. As the candle is blown out, the Light can be sent out to where it is needed, as when working alone.

- Before closing the meeting, the group should carry out the Closing-down Procedure, Chapter 5, pages 56–7. This could be led by the chosen leader.

The reflection time can be used to make notes, or illustrate the experience in some way. It allows the group to log their experience and learning, chart the energies they have been working with and ground the experience, giving the mind time to absorb what has happened.

Working with the injured and dying

You have heard a news item about the dire situation of people in a certain war zone. When this item comes up on TV, there are close-up pictures of the injured, including women and children. These scenes become imprinted on your mind. You decide that you will include them in your next Distant Healing session. You make sure that you will be able to maintain a calm state and that you will be able to work unconditionally. When you sit to work and find yourself needing to do this in the advanced (astral) way, your session could go something like the following.

EXERCISE 51
Sending out to the injured and dying – astral level healing

First check your mental and emotional response to the situation. Your healing request should be unconditional. Do not decide in advance what you think should happen. This allows decisions to be made at the level of the Higher Self. Remember, healing energy, like prayer, travels at the level of the intentional thought.

Healing Light will always help the dying to pass over. As with earlier situations, this Light will also be needed by the rescue team and those who were witnesses to what happened. So be prepared to go with the flow of your guidance and make a note of your experience later.

- Make sure that you will not be interrupted in any way. Prepare and dedicate your working space. Attune yourself, light your candle and dedicate the work. Ask to be used as a channel for healing, and to be guided by your Higher Self (soul). You will look forward to being directed by this source (whether or not you will be doing any Distant Healing at the astral level).

- Sit with your feet flat on the floor with your hands, palms up, on your thighs or in your lap. The hands should not overlap or touch. (In astral work it is essential for the palm centres to remain active, hence the palms-up position of the hands.) Use the breath to calm and relax the body. Let go of any worries or anxieties with the out-breath, through the open mouth. When you feel attuned, close your mouth and breathe normally. Check that your body is

exercise continues ▶

relaxed, including the back of the neck, the shoulders and pelvis. Sit in the silence for a few moments.

- Close your eyes to aid concentration and allow the faces and bodies of the dead and injured to come to mind again. Check that you can make your request without adding your own opinions or judgement.

- Wait quietly and patiently to see if you become aware that a subject is in front of you.

- If you have been 'taken' to the person, or the person has been 'brought' to you, you will sense this. This becomes easier when you relax and accept that it is possible for this to happen. You will also be able to sense whether the adult person, child or baby is lying or sitting in front of you and how the body is orientated.

- Mentally make sure that you are comfortably orientated to carry out what needs to be done. Allow your intuitive guidance to help you sense where your hands need to go.

- If this is what is needed, you will feel healing energy leave your hands, or whatever sign tells you that you are working. Keep them in the same position until you feel a change in the flow of energy, which could be sensed as a marked decrease, or falling off, in intensity. The signal is that all, or part, of the healing is complete.

- Wait for your guidance to see if you need to give healing elsewhere. The energetic activity in your hands is confirmation that this is not taking place in your imagination. A person with developed perceptions would be able to sense or 'see' what was going on and confirm that you were working this way.

- When you have completed your work with the subject, mentally thank them. Now take a full breath and, as you exhale, surround them with a protective sphere of light. This may be done mentally or by raising your arms and moving your hands gently to make a sphere around the astral body in front of you (Figure 21, page 120).

exercise continues ▶

- When there is another subject to work with, first make sure that the one you were working on is no longer in front of you. Visualise clearing silver light washing over your upraised palms. You can now proceed to the next subject. Take a short pause if you feel the need.

- Follow the same procedure as before. Finally, break your link with the last subject by clearing your hands.

- When you have completed your work, blow out the candle. This can be done by sending out the light of the candle. Pause for a moment to see if you intuitively feel where it needs to go. As you blow out the candle, say: 'I send the Light out to –.'

- Carry out the Closing-down Procedure outlined in Chapter 5, pages 56–7.

If, during an astral level healing, you sense that you are no longer sitting in your chair, but standing over or by the subject, this tells you that you have travelled to them. Keep relaxed and proceed as described above. You are quite safe and can move out of this state whenever you like.

This way of working requires intense, but relaxed, concentration. Because of this, I recommended earlier that you start working this way with one subject at a time, with an aim of no more than six in any one session, unless guided otherwise. You need to feel totally comfortable and build up your confidence so that you do not get tired by the level of focused effort needed to work this way. In the case above, I am assuming that you have achieved this level of confidence. Keep a note of what happens in your journal.

By the time you have used both baseline and advanced techniques with the second group of the crucial world issues, you may have a feeling that the work resonates for you in a special way. Perhaps you would like to specialise in this area. Your Distant Healing journal will give you clues about this.

You have discovered that there is a great deal of work to be done in this field and all the other fields of work that we have covered on your healing journey so far. Life presents us with many difficult and scary situations but, in the midst of them, and surrounding them, is the eternal beauty of the world. There is humour, courage, determination to accentuate the positive, and look for the Light; and there are always moments of wonder.

On this journey, you are responsible for you. Distant Healing emphasises that there are two sides to life, not just the negative. Take steps to keep your life in balance. It is important to look after yourself, to keep yourself well, to enjoy life. This will ensure that you keep your healing channel open and in prime condition. In the final chapter we will look at how to do this. All good endings have a surprise – and I have one for you.

Part Four

Chapter 14

A way of being

The heart centre – taking care of the divine dream

In this final chapter we revisit the heart centre. Distant Healing begins in this centre because it is the focal point of the divine dream of incarnation – of the total human being. As we near the end of our work together, this may seem obvious, but how this came about is one of the wonders of the human being.

Human birth is the grounding of the divine dream, the earthing of the Light of Oneness. We know that living beings, the planet and the cosmos on which they depend, are facets of Oneness. Because Oneness means that if any part of the whole is suffering then every part experiences that suffering, to take care of the divine dream is a responsibility that is at the core of the Distant Healing agenda.

With their understanding of spiritual reality, indigenous and shamanic cultures have always accepted that restoring balance and harmony at the subtle levels is as necessary as restoring physical health and well-being. Distant Healing moves between both of these worlds, as well as being in them, and so complements (and is not an alternative to) allopathic medicine, and all therapeutic practice, because it operates on all levels of our being.

The creative role of the heart centre

In Chapter 3, I described how the Light being that we are needs a series of vehicles, or 'bodies', in order to travel on the various levels, culminating in the physical body. The significance for Distant Healers is the crucial role that the heart centre plays in this embodiment process.

Once the spiritual intention has been put in place, the physical body is prepared through the activation of the etheric template. As the incoming spiritual force moves towards physicality, it first becomes embodied in a spirit body. The energy of the spirit body moves to meet the incoming spiritual force and the two merge at what we know as the heart centre. The spirit body, with its heart centre, is the soul or Higher Self. From here, the spiritual force takes on a number of other bodies, or vibrating patterns of energy. Spirit has become embodied at a mental, emotional, etheric and physical level. Each energy pattern is vibrating at a rate lower than the incoming spiritual force, becoming progressively slower until the physical level is reached. At each stage of embodiment, the energy of the next 'body' merges with the spiritual force at the heart centre. Thus, the heart centre is where we hear the voice of the Higher Self, often in the form of feelings.

Maintaining the channel

Maintaining your own healing channel is the same thing as understanding and maintaining your heart centre. When the focus of your attunement is the heart centre, it ensures that you engage with the indwelling spiritual force, and your mental and emotional intention is sent out at this level. Looking after your heart centre, then, is the key to maintaining your healing channel.

Once a week, look into your heart centre in a calm, observant way. Acknowledging that this is the place of the soul, ask yourself if your heart centre is a combination of serene temple and lively workshop, or is it a place of confinement and frustration? Perhaps you have a sense already, but you can make an accurate assessment with the next exercise.

EXERCISE 52

Assessing the state of the heart centre

- Sit quietly where you will not be disturbed. Put one hand over

exercise continues ▶

your heart centre. Does it feel warm or cold, soft or hard, alive or struggling to live?

- Imagine that you can see into your heart centre. Visualise that it has two equal halves, each with two chambers, somewhat like your physical heart. The left half receives energy, receives life; the right half gives out energy, gives out to life.

- You need to have a fully functioning heart. Take a look at the left half. Ask your heart centre: How am I closed to receiving love? Wait for the response.

- To be fully receptive you need to be open to life, feel good about yourself, and clear about your choices. When you feel closed, defensive and wanting to avoid painful situations, or be protected from them, you need to loosen up and discover what really matters to you. When difficulties come your way, the first step is to accept them. You will be able to use Distant Healing as your next step.

- When you feel indifferent about things, full of doubts and unable to make choices, the receptive half of your heart centre is asking you to conserve energy, gather your strength and wait patiently for clarity and inspiration. Recognise these energies when they appear so that you can receive them.

- Now look at the right half of your heart centre. Ask your heart centre: How do I stop myself giving love? Wait for the response.

- To be fully able to give out energy as a healing and vitalising force, you need to be able to sense the inner strength that makes you wholehearted in what you do. When you feel half-hearted and apathetic, you are in the wrong place. This could be the wrong physical, emotional, mental or spiritual place, or a combination of them. It's time to remove yourself from the situation. Patiently hold on to your own space until you feel the energies of interest and excitement returning.

exercise continues ▶

- When you realise that you are not being authentic, not being the real you, you have uncovered a lack of courage (the power of the heart, which is actually a form of love). Again, look into yourself and decide what really matters to you, what seems to have 'heart'? Take charge of your energies and put what has heart back into your life. This will unlock courage, and unlock the ability to give and receive love.

Each of the exercises that follow helps towards your goal of achieving a fully functioning heart centre and maintaining the healing channel.

EXERCISE 53

Heart centre breathing

This exercise is excellent for balancing and revitalising the system, especially when working from the heart centre as in Distant Healing.

- Sit comfortably with your feet flat on the ground. Rest your hands on your thighs, palms up (in receptive mode). Breathe normally. Relax your elbows, the back of your neck and the tops of your shoulders. Do this by 'letting go' with each out-breath. Close your eyes if this helps you to concentrate.

- Breathe into the heart centre. As you do so, see a green light there that gets brighter each time you inhale. Allow the green light to fill up the heart centre and move out into the area of the body around it.

- Let your focus move slowly and gently down to the solar plexus centre. See a golden yellow light as you inhale. Allow this light to fill up the centre and the area of the body around it.

- Now let your focus move slowly and gently down to the sacral centre. See a bright orange light as you inhale. Allow this light to fill up the centre and the area of the body around it.

exercise continues ▶

- Let your focus move slowly and gently down to the base centre. See a bright red light as you inhale. Allow this light to fill up the centre and the area of the body around it.

- Return your focus to the heart centre. See the green light awaiting you. Let your focus slowly and gently rise to the throat centre. See a sky-blue light as you inhale. Allow this light to fill up the centre and the areas of the throat, nose and ears.

- Let your focus slowly and gently rise to the brow centre. See a royal-blue or indigo light as you inhale. Allow this light to fill up the centre and the head and eyes.

- Let your focus slowly and gently rise to the crown centre. See a violet light as you inhale. Allow this light to fill up the centre, and cover the top of the head.

- Return your focus to the heart centre. See the green light awaiting you again. Relax and breathe naturally.

This exercise is an excellent antidote to the effects of negative information on the centres (as described in Chapter 9, page 99).

The heart centre is the place of balance for the seven main subtle energy centres. As well as reminding us that our core is the Higher Self, this means that the centre is able to bring balance to *all* the levels of our being. Next is a simple exercise in which the heart centre plays the role of balancing the body energies.

EXERCISE 54

Balancing body energies

This exercise can be done anywhere as long as you have a place to lie down. As well as balancing the body energies, the exercise relaxes and refreshes the system.

exercise continues ▶

- Loosen the clothing and make sure there is no constriction around your neck. Lie down in a firm, comfortable place, with the head supported. The legs should be a little apart, with the arms by the sides of the body.
- Take three full breaths, letting go of tension as you exhale. Breathe naturally and 'let go' of the body. Focus on the heart centre with the eyes open.
- Remain relaxed but alert, without allowing yourself to drift off. Let your body find its own relaxed position. Listen to the body as it finds its own balance. Notice how areas of tension relax. Some of your limbs may move slightly.
- Maintain your focus on the heart centre.
- After about 15 minutes, the body's energies have become balanced. When this occurs, a tingling sensation or feeling of internal lightness may be sensed all over the body. Remain lying in this position for as long as you need to.
- You will feel refreshed. Before getting up, give thanks for the body's ability to refresh itself in this way.

Greeting the day

Keeping your healing channel open means being conscious of your alignment with the sacred and you can soon make this a part of your daily routine. There are numerous ways of starting the day with this in mind. I like to start my day by acknowledging the Sun as a symbol of the Light. The next exercise promotes your sensitivity to the natural cycles of giving and receiving.

The seven breaths of greeting symbolise the seven directions of East, South, West, North, Above, Below and Within.

EXERCISE 55

The Seven Breaths of Greeting

If possible, practice this exercise outside.

- Face the direction of the dawn, the place of the rising sun, standing or sitting. Use your breath to relax the body. Become aware of your feet and their contact with the ground. Feel your connection to the Earth.

- Give thanks for the previous night. Be aware that the source of energy, and the promise of each day, is within you.

- Feel the air around you. Become aware of your breath and the fresh air entering your nostrils and your lungs. Note how your whole body enjoys the breath of the new day.

- Now, as you breathe slowly and naturally, raise your arms as if you are lifting them up to the sun.

- In this position of thanks and greeting take seven deep breaths down into the abdomen. As you inhale, visualise the life force in the air moving into the various parts of your body and energy field in the following sequence:

- With the first breath, visualise the life force moving down the length of your spine, filling it with life and relaxing the muscles of your back.

- With the second breath, take the life force down into your pelvis and legs, allowing it to relax the muscles of these parts.

- With the third breath, take the life force into the shoulders and arms, allowing it to relax the muscles.

- With the fourth breath, let the life force fill the head and neck, relaxing the neck.

- With the fifth breath, let the life force fill the organs of the abdomen, relaxing the abdominal muscles.

exercise continues ▶

- With the sixth breath, let the life force fill the chest and heart centre, relaxing the muscles of the chest.

- With the seventh breath, let the life force fill your whole energy field, harmonising and balancing the energies within it.

- Enjoy this state of harmony for a few moments before moving off.

You can vary how you direct the seven breaths according to your needs on any particular day. For example, you may need to focus more energy on a specific part of the body. If you are able to practise the exercise outside, notice the world around you as you calmly take your breaths. Feel your sacred connection with life being renewed. Acknowledge the other life forms that may be present.

Honouring food

Communicating with your body about food can be a revelation. We rarely ask it what it *needs* and demand that it copes with what we want, when and how we want it. We are not concerned how it feels when we rush to eat, or eat without caring what we put in our mouth. The next meal may be the right time to communicate with it.

Because your food has been part of a living plant or animal, handled by different people and machinery, transported and packaged, it contains a range of vibrations, some of which are not compatible with yours. Blessing your food thanks it, clears it, and brings its energies into alignment with your own. Using your hands in a sacred manner to bless food enhances the subtle energy structures of the palms.

EXERCISE 56

Blessing and thanking food

- When you are going to eat or drink something, first hold your

exercise continues ▶

hands over it to see if your body really needs it. If you sense that it does not, honour your intuitive awareness and the body's friendly message by not consuming it. Of course, this process should ideally begin in the shop!

- All food and drink can be honoured through your remembrance of the hand-heart link. Use your hands to bless and thank your food and drink before consuming them.

Mealtimes should always be harmonious. Your body will tell you that food should always be eaten with enjoyment and never with anxiety about what it is made of, and so on. Blessing your food has taken care of this, so go ahead and enjoy your food as a gift from the planet. Thank those who grow and prepare it for you, as well as those working in factories where the meal has been manufactured (when this is the case).

Getting together, celebrating and eating with others are wonderful ways of sharing food. When you have reached this point in the book, why not decide how you could celebrate your achievement with a party!

Distant Healing support energies – the third challenge

Distant Healing emphasises the positive while working with the negative. Your journey with this book has shown you the huge variety of situations that need the benefits of healing. But you will have also noticed how an important aspect of Distant Healing is its supportive role.

My surprise for you is that we can go further in this supportive role, that there is actually a third challenge for Distant Healers today: to send out to those people and organisations that are doing constructive work for the whole – whether human, animal, plant or environmental, and to situations where these positive activities are taking place. As it does for the teams involved in rescue and care, the energy of Love will help and support, as well as heal. Secondly, the positive energy field that you will help to create, around those people and situations, will attract what is needed. As in all your work, Distant Healing support energies must be sent unconditionally. You do not need to decide what are the 'good' things and who are the most 'deserving'.

An attitude of open-heartedness is ensured by your being aware of what comes into your orbit, of what is presented to you, because you are the person to deal with it. Life is coming towards you every moment. Be receptive and take it as it comes, giving thanks for it. Giving thanks completes the energy circle.

To get used to working with this third challenge, let's take a typical example, which is one of many possibilities.

EXERCISE 57
Sending out to a project

You hear about a certain project which is doing work to help underprivileged people. The project resonates with you and you would like to send out Distant Healing Support energies.

- Make sure the phone is disconnected and that you will not be disturbed. Attune both your work space and yourself as before.

- You may wish to light a candle as a symbol of the Light of the Source. If so, dedicate it to the work and any helpers you might have in the spiritual realms. Give thanks that you have been given the opportunity to send out the Light of Support.

- Bring your focus to your heart centre. As you inhale, visualise this centre filling with the Light. With the next breath, the Light fills your chest.

- Ask for the Light to be sent out to the project you have in mind. You can say aloud or in your mind: 'I ask for support to be sent to (name the project and all those working for it).'

exercise continues ▶

- Give thanks and rest assured that the project and project workers have received the Distant Healing Support energies they need. Sit quietly with your experience.

- When you have completed your work, blow out the candle. This can be done by sending out the light of the candle. Pause for a moment and see if you intuitively feel where it needs to go. This is usually the first thing that comes to mind. As you blow out the candle, you could say: 'I send the Light out to all that is beautiful in our world.'

- Once you have closed your session, you have handed over the list to higher powers.

By now, you won't be surprised if exercises like that take you into advanced-level mode, if this is what is needed. Go with the flow of the energies. Practice will soon get you used to the idea that you can send support and goodwill as easily as you can send healing help.

The group scenario will be very similar to the one you have already practised. If the group agrees, Distant Healing Support can be part of your work together. Attunement and your focus in the heart centre will always honour the fact that Love is unconditional.

Being aware of beauty

Beauty tells us about soul. Our connection to beauty nourishes us at a deep level. Take time to notice the beauty around you and in Nature and to be with whatever (and whomever) you find beautiful. This is the perfect antidote to noticing the negative and constantly dealing with what needs healing.

Finally, here is an exercise to honour beauty and your whole experience of the natural world. It is a fun thing to do either alone or with your Distant Healing group.

EXERCISE 58

Honouring beauty and the natural world

If possible, practise this exercise outdoors. Take yourself somewhere you find especially beautiful. If you can't get out, study a beautiful photo or picture first. If you are unable to take up the bodily positions described, the exercise may still be done through your mental intention and visualisation.

- Lie down with your back touching the ground. Have your legs slightly apart, arms relaxed by your sides, hands with palms up. Relax your body and breathe naturally.

- Now, being aware of the ground, and the Earth that nurtures you, breathe in the Light through the whole top surface of your body. Take your time with this exercise.

- Lying on your back, be aware that every plant, with its roots in the soil, pushes up into the light with its growing tip. Being aware of your connection to the plant world, carefully breathe the Light into the tips of your fingers and toes.

- Still lying on your back, be aware of the waters of the Earth and the creatures that live in them.

- Turn over and rest comfortably on the front of your body, with your arms bent at the elbows and palms resting on the ground in line with your head. Being aware of the creatures that travel over the Earth, breathe the Light into the whole back surface of your body.

- Being aware of the creatures that live under the Earth, breathe the Light into the whole back surface of your body again.

- When you feel ready, stand up and fold your arms, across your heart centre, then slowly open them, completely extending your arms on a level with your shoulders. Being aware of all the beings that fly, breathe the Light into your heart centre.

exercise continues ▶

- Relax your arms by your sides. Check that your feet are a shoulder-width apart with your knees gently flexed. Slowly raise your arms, with the palms upwards, to form a Y-shape. Being aware of the trees, breathe the Light into your palms. Be aware of your 'branches', your 'trunk' and your 'roots'.

- Relax your arms by your sides again. Spend a few moments with this experience.

- In a group situation, this would be a good time to have a group hug!

Personal energetic health and hygiene

As long as you follow the guidelines of the book, you will learn to function as a Distant Healer safely, effectively and with confidence.

Looking after your heart centre is as important as looking after your physical heart. Similarly, your personal energetic health and hygiene are as necessary as keeping your body clean, flexible and vigorous. This is maintained by carrying out the clearing, closing down and protection exercises whenever you have concluded your work; before going to sleep; before going out and mixing with other people and before a leisure or sporting activity (see in Chapter 5, page 56). You may be surprised at how open your subtle energy system is after reading or working with this book!

Keeping a journal

Your Distant Healing journal will act like the best friend you need to confide in on your healing journey. As well as a useful record of what happens and charting your development as an energy worker, it is the place for other relevant comments, insights, dream material and anything else that has a bearing on your work. But words may not always be the way you want to log your experiences. Sometimes a drawing, painting or some other kind of creative work will be far more expressive.

Looking back on your journal can be a rewarding experience. You will have a fascinating personal record that shows how you engaged with *The Distant Healing Handbook*. You may discover new abilities, new possibilities and new friends.

I thank you for the work that you will do to help *all our relations*.

Glossary

Acupuncture: an energy therapy that uses the activation, by special metal needles, of energy points on the etheric meridians; common to Chinese Medicine.

Allopathic: contemporary medicine, particularly medicine using drugs in the treatment of illness.

Aura: the total energetic emanation of the human being, including the physical, etheric and other energy zones. The human energy field.

Breath: the main way that we take in the life force, therefore considered as sacred by many cultures from ancient times. A *kahuna* healer from Hawaii told me that the mystical meaning behind the greeting *aloha* (in the presence of the breath of life) is the wish to share *ha* (sacred breath).

Chakra: now a common term for a subtle energy centre. From Sanskrit, *chakram*, 'wheel'. The whirling vortex of energy looks somewhat like a turning wheel.

Distant Healing: healing when the subject is at a distance from the healer. When capitalised, refers to the particular form and techniques outlined in this book.

Earth: when capitalised, refers to our planet, from the Distant Healing point of view, as a being in its own right.

Earth Family: the other beings that share the Earth with us.

Energy: in Distant Healing, a force directed by, and emanating from, the Source. Spirit is the energy of the Source. Compared with this level of energy, the physical has a vastly lower frequency.

Energy centre: a subtle structure, detected in the etheric body, designed to allow the flow of subtle energies into and out of the human energy field. The subject of Chapter 8, pages 81–98.

Etheric: the energetic level next to the physical at which energy vibrates at a higher frequency. Acts as the bridging zone between the physical and the subtle and is the support system for the physical body. From the Ancient Greek term *ether*, which referred to the upper regions of the atmosphere, or heaven. Seers of the time had witnessed that, on passing over, people carried on being in their 'heavenly' or etheric body.

Higher Self: the human soul; the indwelling spiritual force of the human being.

Life force: the vital energy, essential to life, conducted by the subtle energy system. The same as *prana* (Sanskrit), *qi* (Chinese) and *ki* (Japanese).

Light: when capitalised, another word for the Source, Oneness (which some call God). An aspect of spiritual energy. A force that encourages healing and enlightenment.

Love: when capitalised, another word for the Source, Oneness. A force that encourages healing and integration.

Meridian: a channel of subtle energy conduction in the etheric body.

Oneness: when capitalised, another word for the Source (which some call God). A term which describes the sacred unity of all that is.

Patient: a conventional therapeutic term which simply distinguishes the person being helped from the healer.

Personality: the self; the physical consciousness of the self that tends to see itself as separate from all that is: the natural world and the Source, or Oneness.

Polarity balance: the energy systems of living things, including humans, have two aspects or polarities: the receptive (often erroneously termed the 'feminine') and the emissive (often erroneously termed the 'masculine'). The possibility of receiving and giving out energy ensures its cyclic nature. Human health and well-being depends on maintaining a balance between the two energy streams. Whether or not this is the case affects the rest of the Earth and the Earth Family.

Qi Gong: the Chinese system of exercises where breath and movement are used to enhance the intake of *qi*, the life force.

Self: see **Personality** above.

Source: when capitalised, another term for Oneness, which some call God, the Creator. The source of all energies.

Subtle energy: when used in this book, energy vibrating at a higher frequency than physical matter. Such energy, travelling at a velocity beyond the speed of light, behaves in very different ways to those physical energies at present known to most science (see William Tiller in Further Reading and Web Resources, pages 197 and 200).

Subtle energy medicine: any therapy that works primarily with the subtle energy system to bring balance and/or harmony to the subject. Distant Healing is such a healing modality.

Subtle energy system: the co-ordinated system of the etheric body, comprising the energy centres and their etheric network links and the other zones of the energy field.

Further Reading

Angelo, Jack, *Your Healing Power: a comprehensive guide to channelling your healing energy*, Piatkus Books, 1994/2007

Angelo, Jack, *Hands-On Healing*, Rochester, Vermont, Healing Arts Press, 1997

Angelo, Jack and Angelo, Jan, *The Spiritual Healing Handbook: How to develop your healing powers and increase your spiritual awareness*, Piatkus Books, 2007

Arrien, Angeles, *The Four-Fold Way: Walking the Paths of the Warrior, Teacher, Healer and Visionary*, New York, HarperSanFrancisco, 1993

Barnes, Simon, 'No Island Is An Island', *Birds* (magazine of the RSPB, Royal Society for the Protection of Birds), *vol. 21, no. 4*, 2006

Dossey, Larry, *Healing Words: The Power of Prayer and the Practice of Medicine*, New York, HarperSanFrancisco, 1993

Dossey, Larry, *Healing Beyond the Body: Medicine and the Infinite Reach of the Mind,* Boston and London, Shambhala, 2001

Gerber, Dr Richard, *Vibrational Medicine*, Santa Fe, New Mexico, Bear & Company, 1988/96

Gerber, Dr Richard, *Vibrational Medicine for the 21st Century*, Piatkus Books, 2000

Krippner, S., and Welch P., *Spiritual Dimensions of Healing*, New York, Irvington Publications, 1992

Lovelock, James, *Gaia: A New Look at Life on Earth*, Oxford and New York, Oxford University Press, 1979

McElroy, Susan Chernak, *Animals as Teachers and Healers*, New York, New Sage Press, 1996; Rider, 1997

Maclean, Dorothy, *To Honor the Earth*, New York, HarperSanFrancisco, 1991

Margulis, Lynn, *The Symbiotic Planet: A New Look at Evolution*, New York, Basic Books, 1998

Pearl, Dr Eric, *The Reconnection*, New York and London, Hay House, 2001

Pecci, Ernest F., and Tiller, William A. *Science and Human Transformation: Subtle Energies, Intentionality and Consciousnss*, Walnut Creek, California, Pavior Publishing, 1997

Suzuki, David, and Knudtson, Peter, *Wisdom of the Elders*, New York and London, Bantam Books, 1992

Tiller, William A., *What Are Subtle Energies?*, Journal of Scientific Exploration, vol. 7, no. 3, 1993

Tiller, William A., Dibble, Walter, and Kohane, Michael, *Conscious Acts of Creation*, Walnut Creek, California, Pavior Publishing, 2001

Walsch, Neale Donald, *Communion With God*, Hodder & Stoughton, 2000

Wilcox, Joan Parisi, *Keepers of the Ancient Knowledge: the Mystical World of the Q'ero Indians of Peru*, London and Boston, Massachusetts, Element Books, 1999

Web Resources

www.alternative-therapies.com
Website of *Alternative Therapies in Health and Medicine* magazine (US).

www.caduceus.info
Website of *Caduceus* magazine – 'healing for people, community and planet' (UK).

www.circleofcompassion.net
Website of Circle of Compassion; 'exploring peaceable choices for the planet and all who share it' (US).

www.contemplativemind.org
Website of the Center for Contemplative Mind in Society (US).

www.dosseydossey.com
Official website of Dr Larry Dossey, who has written extensively on the power of intention and intentional prayer.

www.ecolo.org
Ecological website with section endorsed by Professor James Lovelock.

www.hayfoundation.org
Website of Hay Foundation work.

www.issseem.com
Website of the International Society for the Study of Subtle Energies and

Energy Medicine – a meeting place for scientists, mystics and energy practitioners.

www.jackangelo.com
Official website of Jack Angelo – writer and teacher in the fields of subtle energy medicine, natural spirituality and world spiritual traditions.

www.nccam.nih.gov
Official website of the National Center for Complementary and Alternative Medicine (US).

www.nfsh.org.uk
Website of the National Federation of Spiritual Healers. Leading non-denominational teaching and lobbying organisation – with international links (UK).

www.noetic.org
Website of the Institute of Noetic Sciences (IONS). Founded in 1973, IONS has a number of projects involving distant healing and intentional prayer and an extensive bibliography of scientific studies on distant healing (US).

www.realityshifters.com
Website 'for those who know (or are beginning to suspect) that our thoughts and feelings shift reality'. Information on studies about distant healing (US).

www.resurgence.org
Website of *Resurgence* magazine – linking ecology, spirituality, art and culture (UK).

www.rspb.org.uk
Website of the Royal Society for the Protection of Birds – an organisation also dedicated to environmental protection in general.

www.spiritualityhealth.com
Website of *Spirituality And Health* magazine (US).

www.thereconnection.com
Website of Dr Eric Pearl's work.

www.tillerfoundation.com
Website of Professor William Tiller's work.

www.wholistichealingresearch.com
Website of Wholistic Healing Research, hosted by leading researcher Dr Daniel Benor.

Index

Page numbers in *italics* refer to illustrations

Above (direction) 184
accepting feelings 106–107, 111
accessing body secrets 109
acupuncture 34, 96, 193
Adam 50
addressing the work space 47–49
adrenal glands 42, 87, 105
adrenaline 42
advanced Distant Healing 113–129, 174
ageing, fear of 105
air 133, 138, 141–142, 149, 157
'all our relations' (*mitákuye oyásin*) 95, 192
aloha 193
allopathic medicine 179, 193
Ancient Greeks 30
Andes 135
animals 28, 49, 51, 52, 68, 129, 133, 149, 167, 186
   as healers 155–156
   as teachers 155–156
   dying 162–163
   working with 155–163
Arizona 92
arthritis 91
assessing the heart centre 180–182
astral
   body 115
   travelling 115
astral level 115
   healing 117–128, *119*, 153, *153*, 158–160, 172–174
   Healing Circle 122–128, *123*
attitudes
   negative 104
   positive 51, 103

attention 157, 164
attraction, law of 16, 52
attunement 5, 12, 16, 17–18, 36–37, 41, 44, 47, 49, 53, 94, 99, 102, 144, 180, 189
aura 30, 193
autonomic nervous system 42
awareness 17, 134, 187
   intuitive 93, 94
   psychic 93, 94

balance 71, 78, 87, 88, 91, 95, 99, 110, 134, 135, 136, 137, 144, 175, 179, 182, 183, 194
   polarity 78
balancing 36, 47
   body energies 183–184
Barnes, Simon 133
base centre 33, 58, 71, *82*, 87–88, 90, 91, 95, 96, 104, 105, 138, 139, 183
baseline practice 51–60, 61–63, 174
beauty 189, 190–191
Below (direction) 184
bereavement 14, 82, 128
birds 155, 156
Birds 133
birth 41, 128, 138, 179
blessing food 155, 186–187
blockage, energetic 82, 92, 106, 107, 110
blood 43, 97
blue
   royal- 40, 58, 94, 183

sky- 40, 58, 92, 183
body
   awareness 107–109
   consciousness 13
   template 72
bones 74–75
brain 93, 94, 105
bread 149
breath 41, 193
breathing 17, 23, *24*, 36, 39, 41–43, *42*, 45–47, 89, 99, 138, 140, 141, 167, 182–183, 185
   disturbed 42
   full-breath 43–44
   'soft-belly' 44
brow centre 58, 71, *82*, 89, 93–94, 95, 103, 105, 134, 139, 183

cause and effect, law of 13
central channel 33–4, *33*, 71, 72, 81
central nervous system 73
chakra (see also *energy* centres) 34, 193
checking polarity balance 78–80
children 88
choices 181
clearing 36, 37–38, *38*, 47–48, 57, 191
climate 142
   change 166
Closing-down Procedure 56–60, 64, 67, 121, 125, 147–148, 160, 162, 174, 191
clouds 133
colour 47, 58, 95, 156
   blue, royal 40, 58, 94, 183
   blue, sky 40, 58, 92, 183
   green 39, 58, 91, 136, 137, 182, 183
   indigo 40, 58, 94
   orange 39, 58, 88, 182
   pink 109
   red 39, 58, 87, 194
   violet 39–40, 58, 95, 183
   yellow, golden 39, 58, 89, 182
communicating with the elements 137–142
communication 47, 92, 134, 135, 138, 149, 156, 166
communing 134, 151, 156
communing with
   Air 141–142
   animals 156–157

Earth 138–139
Fire 140–141
Water 140
community 61, 165
   global 14
consciousness 49, 50, 73, 91, 105, 113, 114, 133, 134, 135, 143, 163, 165, 166
   body 13
Conversations with God 136
coping strategies 14, 103, 109
cosmos 129, 179
creating
   the Light column 64–67, *66*
   the Light pool 55–56, 162–163
creation 27, 113, 134
creativity 88, 105, 107, 179, 191
Creator 195
crises 129
   global 64, 67
   local 64, 67
   national 64, 67
crown centre 33, 58, *82*, 88, 93, 94–95, 98, 105, 183

database 6, 7
death 14, 41, 73, 114, 128, 160
   fear of 105
depression 94
diaphragm 41–42, 89
difference 165–166
directions, seven 184
disaster situation *169*, 169–171
disrupted
   energy flow 150
   landscape 141–143
   oceans 143
distant healing 4–6, 11
Distant Healing
   advanced 113–129, 174
   Book 51
   (description) 1, 11–12, 15, 193
   support energies 187–189
   (uses) 2, 14, 50
Distant Healing Circle 61, 62–67, 121, 169–171
   astral level 122–128, *123*
disturbed breathing 42
dog 161–162
Dossey, Dr Larry 13

dream experiences 114
drought 166
dying animal 162–163

ear 92, 105, 183
Earth 14, 18, 27, 28, 95, 96, 137, 139, 149, 163, 190, 193, 194
    element 87
    Family 53, 137, 142, 163, 193, 194
    memory 75
earthquake 166
East (direction) 184
economic issues 164
eczema 91
effects of
    negative energies 99–112
    personal feelings 99–112
Einstein, Albert 15
electromagnetic forces 166
elements 133, 134, 142
    earth 87, 133, 138
    energies 133
    fire 133, 138, 140–141
    water 88
emissive energy stream 41, 71, 194
emotions 28, 89
emotional
    energy 28, 81, 99
    intention 180
    level 28, *29*, 30, 35, 180
    reality 113
    response 172
    state 71, 99
    zone 115, *116*
endocrine glands 86, 89, 93, 102, 103, 104
energetic
    blockage 82
    disruption 142–143
    environment 103
    problem 166
    situations 102
energising 36
energy 193
    circuits, skeletal 74, *74*, 78
    circulation 17
    flow 107, 110, 111, 142, 155, 166, 194
    heavy 37, 92, 97
    medicine, subtle 3
    of group 111, 150
    law of 134
    pattern 28, 89, 134, 135, 180
    positive 107, 187
    web repair 142
energy centres (chakras) 17, 34, 56, 67, 102, 103, 104, 106, 115, 194, 195
    regulating 58
    seven main *33*, 39–40, 58, 72, 81, *82*, 86, 91, 95, 183
energy field 28, *29*, 31–32, 36, 37–38, 39, 56, 60, 93, *116*, 185–186, 195
    universal 12, 36
    work space 47
energy stream
    emissive 41, 71, 194
    'feminine' 41, 194
    'masculine' 41, 194
    receptive 41
engaging with
    the plant world 151
    your landscape 143
environment 7, 14, 129, 149
    working with 133–148
    environmental
    challenge 144
    crisis 135–136
    devastation 155
    healing 142
    organisations 136
    pollution 155
    problems 137, 166
    subjects 136
    work with group 148
ether 194
etheric 28–30, 114, 115, 194
    body *33*, 33, 34, 71, 72, 81, 194
    level 180
    template 93, 180
    zone 115, *116*
ethnic groups 165
Eve 50
exercises 7, 8, 129
existential problems 105
expression 92
eyes 93, 105, 183

face 93
family issues 164
famine 166

feelings 89, 95, 98, 99–112, 113, 180
    accepting 106–107, 111
    working with 109–112
feet 87
female 87
'feminine' energy stream 41, 71, 72, 194
Findhorn community 134
fire (element) 133, 138, 140–141
fly 156
focus 17
food 135, 136, 142, 155, 186–187
    blessing 155, 186–187
    honouring 186
    production 149–150
forehead 93
forest 153
    fire 134
full-body relaxation 45–47
full-breath breathing 43–44

Gaia 137
Gaia: A New Look at Life on Earth 137
gall bladder 89
garden 133, 149, 152
gender 87, 165
Gerber, Dr Richard 115
gland
    endocrine 86, 89, 93, 102, 103, 104
    pineal 94, 103
    pituitary 93, 105
    thymus 87, 90, 103, 105
    thyroid 92, 105
global 144, 145, 150
    community 14, 165
    crises 64, 67
    healing 68
God 194, 195
gravity 166
Great Spirit 156
green 39, 58, 91, 136, 137, 182, 183
    agenda 136–137
greeting the day 184
grief 87, 102
grounding 58, 98, 139
group 8, 50, 61, 111, 129, 152, 163, 189
    energy 111, 150
    environmental work 148
    experience 100–102
    work with plants 154

ha 193
hand–heart energy circuit 97–98, 187
hands 20–26, 87, 90, 91, 98
Hanina ben Dosa 11
harmonising 47
healing
    channel 180–191
    circle 61–68
    global 68
    hands 20–26
    instinct 2, 4–5, 11
    indigenous 6
    journey 6, 191
    Light 55, 62
    list 51, 98
    self- 44
healing energy 3, 11–13, 16, 17, 36, 48, 49, 53, 98, 111, 150, 172
    column 53
    pool 53
Healing Triangle *12*, 19, 49, 153, 158
heart 16, 20, 51, 74, 90, 97, 191
heart centre 17, 18, 19, 20, 33, 48, 58, *82*, 87, 88, 90–92, 95, 102, 103, 105, 106, 111, 112, 113, 129, 137, 138, 141, 156, 179–184, 189, 191
    and creativity 179
    assessing 180–182
    breathing 182–183
heartbeat 42
heavy energy 37, 92, 97
Higher Self (soul) 17, 18, 20, 27, 28, 36, 41, 60, 73, 81, 82, 89, 91, 94, 106, 114, 129, 134, 167, 168, 172, 180, 183, 194
honouring
    beauty 190–191
    food 186
    natural world 190–191
hormones 105
human 129, 133, 134, 136, 142, 149, 179
    energy field 193, 194
hurricane 134
hypothalamus 93, 105

ice 133, 140
illness 14
imbalance 13, 20, 89, 137
immune system 87, 90, 103
incarnation 179

indigenous
    healing 6
    people 134, 136, 143, 144, 179
indigo 40, 58, 94
individual self (personality) 17, 36, 73, 89
Industrial Revolution 136
injustice 92
inner
    child 88
    teacher 149
    vision 135
    voice 149
intelligence 27
intention 11, 13, 20, 49, 52, 106, 113, 138, 168, 172, 180
intuition 20, 39, 48, 61, 89, 95, 103, 105, 109, 114, 134, 154, 162, 167, 187
intuitive
    awareness 93, 94
    development 113
    self 139
islets of Langerhans 89
issues, life 86
Italy 3–4, 117

Jesus 11
journal 7, 8, 37, 121, 139, 163, 174, 191–192
journey
    healing 6
    soul 13, 14, 16, 27
joy 88, 98, 105, 107, 139
justice 92, 105

kahuna 193
ki 194
kidneys 87, 88, 96

lake 133, 140
landscape 49, 51, 133, 139, 142, 143–145, 163, 167
    disrupted 141–143
landslide 134
laogong point 97
larynx 92
law of
    attraction 16, 52
    cause and effect 13
    energy 134

legs 87
life
    issues 86, 128
    journey 114, 160
life force 43, 138, 141, 185–186, 194
Light 48, 53, 54–55, 62, 73, 80, 94, 95, 103, 105, 135, 145, 146, 167, 172, 175, 179, 184, 190, 194
    column 64–67, *66*
    pool 55, 146–147, 162–163
list, healing 51, 53, 98, 101, 102, 122, 125
listening to a tree 152
liver 74, 89
loss 14
Love 35, 112, 113, 164, 187, 189, 194
love 3, 13, 16, 20, 51, 53, 87, 88, 90, 91, 95, 97, 102, 105, 106, 107, 109, 111, 129, 156, 157, 181
lovelessness 90, 106, 112, 157
Lovelock, James 137
lungs 41–42, *42*, 74, 90

Maclean, Dorothy 134, 137
magpie 156
maintaining the healing channel 180–191
male 87
Margulis, Lynn 137
'masculine' energy stream 41, 71, *72*, 194
media 101, 144, 165
medical procedure 128
meditation 44, 56, 60, 125, 128
mental
    body 28
    development 113
    energy 28, 81
    intention 180
    level 13, 28, *29*, 30, 35, 180
    reality 113
    response 172
    state 71
    turmoil 105
    zone 115, *116*
meridians 34, 194
Middle Eastern healers 11
mind 27, 89, 93, 94
mindset, positive 51
mineral world 75, 133, 149, 150

mitákuye oyásin 95, 192
mountain 133

name 52
   vibration 51
Native Americans 47, 95, 135, 138
nature 87, 91, 105, 129, 133, 136, 142, 164, 165
   honouring 190–191
Nature 136, 142, 149, 189
navel 88, 89
negative
   attitudes 104
   energies 99–112
   feelings 112
   thoughts 167
negativity 100, 101, 102
network of consciousness 166–167
North (direction) 184
nose 92, 105, 183

ocean 133, 140
   disrupted 143
Oneness 1, 12, 16, 18, 35, 50, 73, 91, 95, 129, 135–136, 179, 194, 195
operations 14, 128
orange 39, 58, 88, 182
out-of-body experience 112, 114–115
overlighting spirit 134, 151

palm 20–24, 31, 97
   centres 21, 23, 75, *82*, 86, 95, 97, 98, 186
pancreas 89, 104
partner 8, 22–23, 25, 30–32, 75, 111, 117
pelvis 17, 74, 75, 87, 185
personal
   energetic health and hygiene 191
   feelings, effects of 99–112
   power 89
   self (see personality)
   survival 105
personality 17, 28, 36, 89, 95, 194
pets 156, 157
physical
   body 27–28, 33, 35, 72, 80, 88, 93, 95, 102, 103, 106, 112, 114, 138, 180
   level 13, 137, 180
physicality 87

pineal gland 94, 103
pink 109
pituitary gland 93, 105
planet 87, 98, 136, 137, 138, 150, 152, 164, 179
plant world 150
plants 49, 142, 129, 133, 134, 136, 149, 151, 163, 167, 186, 190
   as teachers and healers 149
   group work with 154
   working with 149–155
polarisation of human behaviour 165–166
polarity
   balance 78–80, 194
   channels 71, 72, 78, 95
political issues 164, 165
pollution 136, 143, 155
positive
   energies 107, 187
   feelings 111
   mindset 51, 103
posture 17, 36, 44
   sitting 18
practice, baseline 51–60
prana 43, 194
prayer 168, 172
procedure
   medical 128
   therapeutic 128
protection 191
psychic awareness 93, 94
purification (sweat) lodge 138

Q'ero people 135
qi 43, 97, 194
Qi Gong 96, 97, 194
quantum mechanics 166
Quest for Gaia, The 137

rain 133, 140, 150
rainbow 95
Rainbow Breath 39–40, *40*
readiness 13, 19
receptive 194
   energy stream 41, 71
red 39, 58, 87, 194
regulating the energy centres 58
relaxation 17, 44–47, 99
   full-body 45–47